Our Unsystematic Health Care System, 2nd Edition

Our Unsystematic Health Care System, 2nd Edition

Grace Budrys

ROWMAN & LITTLEFIELD PUBLISHERS, INC.
Lanham • *Boulder* • *New York* • *Toronto* • *Oxford*

ROWMAN & LITTLEFIELD PUBLISHERS, INC.

Published in the United States of America
by Rowman & Littlefield Publishers, Inc.
A wholly owned subsidiary of The Rowman & Littlefield Publishing Group, Inc.
4501 Forbes Boulevard, Suite 200, Lanham, Maryland 20706
www.rowmanlittlefield.com

P.O. Box 317, Oxford OX2 9RU, UK

British Library Cataloguing in Publication Information Available

Library of Congress Cataloging-in-Publication Data Available

ISBN 0-7425-4296-3 (cloth : alk. paper)   ISBN: 978-0-7425-4297-6
ISBN 0-7425-4297-1 (pbk. : alk. paper)

♾™ The paper used in this publication meets the minimum requirements of American
National Standard for Information Sciences—Permanence of Paper for Printed Library
Materials, ANSI/NISO Z39.48-1992.

Contents

Tables

Preface

Much has changed since the first edition of this book was published in 2001. The initial discussion was heavily influenced by the excitement generated by the Clinton health care reform agenda of the early 1990s and attempts to identify factors responsible for its failure. The discussion presented in this edition reflects the shift in national priorities away from domestic concerns to terrorism and defense. The country is now challenged by the problem of a growing number of people who are losing their health insurance at the same time that health care costs are rising rapidly just when government funds are being reallocated to cover wartime expenses. It is even more troubling to find, through public opinion surveys, that Americans would have difficulty coming to any agreement on what we would do to address the increasing rate of uninsurance even if more funds were available. In short, there is a lot to talk about.

For those who are familiar with the first edition, I want to note the changes that I made in this edition. Chapters 10 and 11 are reversed. In the previous edition, the chapter on reform came before the chapter on other countries. That order reflected the fact that the chapter on reform was so closely tied to discussions that took place when the Clinton reform plan was taking shape. This time, I discuss what other countries have been doing about health care over the last few years before considering reform initiatives being debated in this country.

I have also dropped the recommended readings at the end of each chapter. My rationale is that the pace at which information is being made available has been accelerating over the past few years. This is largely the result of evermore information being presented electronically, on the Internet, than was true even a few years ago. Anyone who wishes to learn more about a particular issue can go to the websites of the organizations and publications that I identify in the text. Those sites often suggest related sites. Because the information is constantly being updated with new documents added, I generally do not identify specific website addresses.

In the preface to the first edition, I said that I was an academic but that the book was not written in a conventional academic style. That statement is true of this edition as well. I make this claim because the writing style is unorthodox by academic standards. My intent is to use a conversational style. I hope that you end up feeling that we are having a conversation throughout the book and that the conversation is a rewarding one. In other words, I hope that I answer many of the questions that come up as we "talk." Another reason for saying that this is not a conventional academic book is that I am not aiming to accomplish traditional academic objectives—to extend the frontiers of knowledge in the field, to challenge prevailing explanations, or to impress colleagues with my erudition. Indeed, the text is not addressed to my colleagues. They already know this material. My objective is to explain it to everyone else. What I say here in the preface however, is likely to be more interesting to colleagues rather than other readers.

I am very pleased that I been given the opportunity to update the book and have many people to thank for getting me to this point. I would like to begin by thanking Alan McClare, the executive editor at Rowman & Littlefield, for his readiness to support a second edition of the book and for his steady encouragement throughout every stage leading to publication. I am grateful to the three anonymous reviewers who reviewed my plans for a second edition and their suggestions regarding points of clarification and topics for expansion. I remain indebted to all the people who were responsible for getting the first edition into print, particularly the initial anonymous reviewer who was so generous in his comments. I will always be indebted to Dean Birkenkamp, the executive editor at Rowman & Littlefield when I submitted the initial draft of the manuscript, for his willingness to take a chance on a book that does not use a conventional academic writing style and format. I wish I could express my gratitude to all the people who have read the book, my students, professors who have used it, and everyone else who has communicated with me to tell me what they like about the book. Finally, my husband, Dan Lortie, deserves special thanks for his willingness to listen to and read early drafts of chapters. My initial drafts tend to be more scathing regarding the failures of our system than they end up being after he reads them. His calming influence has made the writing a lot less vituperative and a lot easier to read.

Introduction to the Health Care System as a Social Institution

In an anecdote popular on the conference circuit, an American health policy analyst who has ascended to heaven asks God, "Will there ever be universal health insurance coverage in the United States?" "Perhaps," sighs God, "but not in my lifetime."

Uwe Reinhardt Ph.D.
Health Affairs, web exclusive
October 23, 2003

Our challenge is huge and growing bigger each year. The time to act is now. There are no easy answers and tough choices will be required. When undertaking reform, the Congress should consider its own Hippocratic oath to "do no harm." Specifically, do not make the long-range financing imbalance worse.

David Walker
Comptroller General of the United States
Government Accountability Office (GAO)
January 13, 2004

This book is about the U.S. health care delivery system. Its main purpose is to explain how the health care system came to look the way it does. While the roots of our health care delivery arrangements could be traced to the earliest period of recorded history, this book aims to address more recent developments concentrating on the twentieth century with most attention directed to the last few decades plus the early years of the twenty-first century. The discussion begins by examining the thinking that led to especially important innovations—that is, policies, programs, and organizations. It goes on to trace what happened once the innovations took effect — in other words, to examine how things evolved once people started creating the organizations needed to implement the newly established policies and programs. Finally, the book outlines the thinking underlying current debates regarding what constitutes the basic problem confronting the health care delivery system and the solutions that would produce the greatest benefit. Whose "thinking"? you might ask. The views expressed by a range of participants and other interested parties, including the general public, policy experts, and occupational or organizational representatives. The quotes at the beginning of each chapter provide a sample of what various people in our society have to say about our health care arrangements. I suspect that these quotes will become more meaningful in hindsight, so I suggest that you reread them as you finish each chapter.

The book views the U.S. health care delivery system from a sociological perspective. I try to keep the sociological jargon to a minimum. My aim is to introduce you to four basic sociological concepts, to which I refer periodically throughout the book. Of course, the question then becomes, Why not just talk about the health care system without turning to what some people would say is pretentious academic language? My answer is that I am convinced that individuals need a framework in which to organize all the information they are confronted with when looking at the health care system. This is especially important under present circumstances given that we are being bombarded with wildly differing interpretations of reality by assorted experts as well as other less-informed but adamant onlookers. I have chosen to use a sociological framework because I am a sociologist: it is the perspective through which I see the world, and it really does offer an excellent lens though which a person can better focus on the details in the design of the health care system.

I rely on several sociological concepts. First, I propose to treat the health care system as a social institution. Second, I show how it has been socially constructed. The third and fourth sociological concepts provide two alternative theoretical frameworks for understanding how its performance can be seen from two distinctly different points of view: functionalism and conflict theory. I explain what sociologists mean by "social institution" in this chapter. The other three sociological ideas provide the substance of chapter 2.

SOCIAL INSTITUTION AS A CONCEPT

When sociologists talk about a social institution, they have in mind a range of processes and structures that operate to address a particular social need, which, in this case, is the need for health care services. The term *social institution* is not to be confused with the term *institution*. We may refer to particular organizations, such as the Mayo Clinic, the Harvard Medical School, the Los Angeles County Hospital, as institutions because they are well known and widely respected. When sociologists use the term *social institution*, they are referring to all the organizations with connections to that particular sector of society—in this case, the health care system. Although the nomenclature is somewhat confusing, sociologists had to find a way to refer to multiple organizations operating in connection—thus, "social institution."

Five social institutions are generally recognized by sociologists, at least those who write introductory sociology textbooks. These are

1. *education*, which operates to provide new members of the society with basic skills, integrates people into society, and selects those who are best qualified to go further in their education;
2. *family*, which represents society's views regarding the responsibilities and privileges that accompany marriage, child bearing, and extended kinship;
3. *religion*, which distinguishes the sacred from the profane, provides guidelines for behavior, and helps people express their spirituality;
4. the *economy*, which organizes the production and distribution of goods and services in the society; and
5. *politics*, which is the arrangement that operates to represent the prevailing distribution of power and decision-making authority in society.

Health care delivery arrangements have not been considered from this perspective until recently simply because, historically, they have not attracted as much attention as they have been attracting lately. However, once you begin thinking about it, you can see that the health care delivery system has much in common with other social institutions. It evolved to address a fundamental social need, and it was built on the same foundation as the other social institutions. The building blocks that serve as the foundation on which all social institutions are constructed comprise our basic cultural values, beliefs, traditions, and expectations about the behavior of others. This explains why social institutions are not identical from one society to another. Each society selects from its own stock of distinctive building blocks.

If the reference to building blocks connotes a construction site, then you have inferred the image as intended. Such imagery helps to explain how the health care system came to look the way it does. It has been constructed much as a multigeneration house has, with several owners continuing to remodel and build additions to suit their needs at the time. Sociologists would say that social institutions are "socially constructed," meaning that our health care delivery system was constructed without the aid of any natural, scientific, sacred, or other to-be-discovered set of rules for designing a social institution. The people who built it simply added the blocks they wanted to see included in the structure. Because there are always so many contributors who want to add their bit and because no one has the authority to order or prevent others from doing so, the design of the entity being built is unpredictable—thus, there is no way to know whether it will operate smoothly and efficiently. Since no one has come up with a better approach to building social institutions, this is the way that we will undoubtedly continue to build them, cumbersome and imprecise though they may be.

It is important to realize that the process of building social institutions is never really finished. People are continually engaged in constructing new additions and making adjustments to prevailing arrangements. Whether the resulting structures turn out to be well designed, satisfying, or beneficial to society lies within the eye of the beholder. It is the users and other interested observers who decide how well the institution meets their respective needs or society's needs.

True, most people have little to say about what social institutions look like. However, the choices made and opinions expressed by individuals and groups across the country are ultimately responsible for shaping them. Social institutions generally do not provide interested parties with a regularly scheduled opportunity to evaluate and possibly alter the programs the institution aims to pursue. The exception to this generalization is the political system. It operates with a schedule for voting on the persons and political parties who will govern for a set period of time. The thinking regarding the operations of other social institutions is harder to capture and document, which makes the matter of implementing society's preferences highly uncertain.

To sum up, sociologists conceptualize social institutions first and foremost as human creations. Second, sociologists believe that social institutions represent some degree of consensus regarding society's beliefs about the best approach for fulfilling fundamental social needs. (What is worth considering—and I do so later in this discussion—is whether society is truly satisfied or whether it has been manipulated into believing that it is happy with current arrangements.) Third, sociologists are convinced that social institutions are dynamic rather than static; they change as society's needs and demands change. Social institutions must be maintained, and sometimes they need to be totally rehabilitated, much as physical structures do. Just as rehabilitating is rarely trouble free, the process through which society constructs and alters its social institutions is fraught with unanticipated problems. Altering one part of the structure often requires some other part being shored up; but because the subsequent alteration is unexpected, there is often no contingency plan for its being accomplished.

CONSTRUCTING AND REHABILITATING INSTITUTIONS

A particularly noteworthy characteristic of social institutions is that their operations are under constant scrutiny. In the case of the health care system, active participants (doctors, nurses, patients, insurance company executives) as well as various interested observers (academics, special interest organizations such as the American Association of Retired Persons) continue to issue statements about institutional performance. Vigorous debate about the need for adjustment erupts from time to time.

The social institution of education provides a good illustration. As I am sure you will agree, public schools receive a fair share of steady criticism, which periodically erupts into more aggressive demands for reform. Someone is always arguing how the schools fail our children and how we can remedy the situation—for instance, raising taxes to support schools, getting rid of teachers who do not teach well, letting a private company operate the schools.

Another example of the scrutiny that social institutions undergo can be seen in the growing number of commentators who have been expressing alarm about the shifting role of religion in society. They say that we should be concerned about both the steady drop in membership among traditional religions and the increase among fundamentalist sects. They argue that this trend brings with it more conservative views, a declining level of tolerance for behavior fundamentalists consider sinful and a growing demand for restricting such behavior. The ongoing battle over how to present sex education in schools, if at all, and whether home schooling is really a good alternative to the traditional classroom are topical examples. In these examples, we can also see two or three social institutions competing to establish control over the schools and schooling. Since it is not clear whose authority and preferences should come first or if the problems they identify really require major changes, the debates and battles continue until enough people in society either take sides or stop listening.

Reaction to reports on the state of the economy provide yet another illustration of how social institutions are shaped by ongoing public debate. A range of questions stand at the center of that debate—for example, are there enough new jobs being created? Are they "good" jobs? Are too many middle-class jobs being "outsourced," that is, exported to other countries? And so on. We have been hearing even more regarding the political realm—more specifically, whether our political leaders are making the right decisions regarding both foreign and domestic policy.

It is during debates of this kind that some critics ultimately proclaim that one of the institutions is failing and that its failure will have cataclysmic effects on society. From the sociological perspective, lamenting the decline of a social institution distorts the issue. It is not the social institutions that fail; it is society that fails to update them. Talk about institutional failure indicates that society's beliefs and preferences have changed and that the social institution in question has not adapted and, for that reason, is no longer meeting society's needs as well as it did previously. To the extent that enough people in a society come to the conclusion that a social institution is failing to meet their needs and expectations, or at least not meeting them well enough, someone must decide what to do about it. There are always those who would prefer to have people return to earlier patterns of behavior. Others want to make specific kinds of adjustments in the processes or structures that operate within that social institution. Rarely does anyone suggest total restructuring of an existing social institution.

In the case of health care, the option of returning to earlier patterns is not possible. Both the organizational structures and the public's expectations about health care—indeed, medicine's ability to overcome health problems—have changed too much over the last few decades to allow a return to earlier arrangements. As a result, society has been struggling with proposals aimed at making specific alterations and adjustments in health sector structures and processes, some of which involve minor changes and others that propose radical changes. The debate regarding the need for change in our health care arrangements erupted into the public realm on a number of occasions, most recently during the early 1990s. This is the era when a significant number of Americans decided that the health care system was no longer working as well as it had been and that it required major change. The presidential campaign that resulted in the first-term Clinton victory, in 1992, moved the topic to the center of political debate.

Since societies rarely try to change social institutions all at once, what happened during the early 1990s came close to being revolutionary. Stable Western democracies are not well equipped to handle radical institutional change. The fact that the discussion of proposals, which would have led to total reform of the health care delivery system, got as far as it did is indicative of the level of social concern about the performance of this institution. It showed that a large number of people in this society really did want to see the health care delivery system altered to better meet society's needs; yet, all the effort that went into designing a reform plan simply faded out within a year or so.

The remaining chapters of the book try to explain why changing the system to meet society's expectations turns out to be so difficult. Before we start our discussion, however, I would like to make a few comments that might help in reading this material.

THE ORGANIZATION OF THE MATERIAL TO COME

Let's start with a comment on the title of the book. I continue to refer to the "health care delivery system" even though most people who study health care arrangements, regardless of their perspective, would say that it is inaccurate to call what we have "a system." The term *system* suggests "systematic" and orderly arrangements. Most observers would agree that what we have is far from systematic because there is so much inconsistency across policies and programs from place to place and, therefore, from case to case. Calling it a system simply means that the whole social institution is the object of discussion. Calling it an "unsystematic system" may sound logically inconsistent, but it is more accurate.

There is no other way to discuss what follows with anything but the language that has evolved to address health care delivery issues. Get ready to encounter a fairly large number of new concepts. It's not that they are hard to understand, but they number so many that it is difficult to remember them all. Thus, I try to define each new concept as it becomes central to the discussion.

References present a problem as well. If I were to give credit to everyone whose ideas I rely on, half of every page would be filled with citations. Many people have done a great deal of work that has subsequently become common knowledge, and they should be given credit for moving all of us to this stage. However, that would seriously detract from the flow of the discussion. I provide specific citations to the work of authors whose work stands out for some reason—because it is commonly referenced, it provides very specific quantitative data, or it is particularly assertive.

It is worth noting that the experts in this field argue about the facts. The nature of their arguments deserves careful attention. The experts tend to argue, sometimes in print, about the quality of the research or the data. While most researchers lament not having complete data, they acknowledge that they must work with the data currently available to them. I do that as well: I cite government statistics that represent all Americans, studies that focus on smaller samples and narrower issues, and efforts to bring together related studies. Timeliness is one of the problems that researchers lament most. It is difficult to collect, analyze, and report findings on what is happening right now. Critics sometimes argue that by the time the findings are reported, they are already out of date—and it is not always easy to know whether that is true. In the chapters to follow, we will look at a range of studies—old and new, big and small—recognizing that there will be new research just around the corner that may support or contradict current research. In the end, most reasonable people agree that it is the compilation of research to which we must attend rather than any one set of findings which we find compelling for the moment.

Before we jump into this venture, I have a couple of warnings for you. First, as you become more involved in this discussion—and I do, of course, hope you become very much involved—you will undoubtedly develop opinions about how you would like to see the system work. That's good! When you present your ideas to others, keep in mind that your argument will be far more convincing if you can say why you are taking your position. In other words, try to refrain from sounding as if you are preaching—as in, people *should* take better care of themselves, or there *should* be more health education, or the government *should* do this or that. Telling people what they should do works fine if you are preaching in the pulpit and conveying the word of a Greater Power. If you, as a mere mortal, tell people what they should be doing, you cannot expect listeners to treat what you say seriously. In short, you will be better off developing a strong argument based on facts as opposed to admonitions.

Second, you may become convinced that you know what motivates various participants to take the stance they are taking. Do not expect to get much support for that approach here. Sociologists have little to say about motivations. In private, we may make some guesses about the intent, goals, and expectations that drive the actions of various participants. However, keep in mind that we really do not place much value on such attributions, because we do not believe we can prove that our attributions are right. Sociologists focus on what they can substantiate—how people behave and what they say they believe. To accurately access people's views about a particular topic at a particular time, we must pose the same questions over and over, because people change their minds. We will examine trend data on attitudes, document the actions of various participants, and perhaps even speculate about *why* they believe what they do or act the way they do—but only if we can agree on the fact that we are only guessing about the *why*.

My third request is to ask you not to use the term *socialized medicine* unless you are certain that you are using it accurately. If you are referring to the systems that existed in Eastern European countries formerly affiliated with the Soviet Union, then talking about socialized medicine makes sense. The concept is also correct when applied to the system that exists in the United Kingdom, although knowledgeable persons do not use that label in connection with the U.K. system. If you invoke this concept in discussing what is happening in the United States, it has the effect of making people like me crazy!

Let me explain. To say that something is "socialized" means that the government not only *runs* whatever it is but *owns* all of the "capital" involved and *employs* all of the personnel. Translating that into terms of the health care delivery system means that the government has total control over all the resources—it owns all the buildings (hospitals, doctors' offices, clinics); hires, fires, and pays all the personnel (doctors, nurses, technicians, aides); and assumes all administrative tasks (sets the budget and determines how many people to hire, what services to provide, where the offices should be located). This accurately describes the National Health Service in the United Kingdom. Other countries have a National Insurance System, which is very different.

Countries that have "national health insurance" systems do not own hospitals or offices, nor do they pay the salaries of all health care personnel. In most cases, doctors work on a fee-for-service basis, meaning that they receive a fee for each health care service they provide to every patient. They may be paid directly by the patients, who are then reimbursed by the national health insurance system, or the doctor may simply bill the national health insurance system. Other health care personnel are generally salaried by hospitals or other health care organizations, which are fully or partially funded, but not owned, by the government. Hospitals in the United States receive most of their income through insurance reimbursements. In short, health insurance, whether it is operated by a national system or privately purchased, is nothing more than "an insurance plan." It works very much as car insurance does.

No one is seriously suggesting that the U.S. health care delivery system be socialized. Those who advocate national health insurance are arguing for an insurance plan for all Americans, one a lot like Medicare. After all, Medicare is basically a "national health insurance system" but only for those Americans who are sixty-five years old and over.

So what do people mean when they warn one another about the forthcoming problems if we go along with plans that lead to socialized medicine? To explain their position, they generally say something like, "If the government runs it, it'll be just as bad as the post office or social security." In my experience, people usually end by adding a little knowing "heh, heh, heh" smirk. This is comparable to the other side of the "should" argument. In this case, the smirk is meant to convey the idea that anyone who would suggest government involvement is too stupid to see how foolish that option is.

This does not preclude your arguing that the government is incompetent and should not be administering a national health insurance system. What it does mean is that you must offer some convincing evidence demonstrating the government's incompetence, and make explicit how a health insurance plan would lead to problems similar to those affecting the postal service or the social security system and how the two are alike. The same is true for those who wish to argue that a government-sponsored health insurance system is the best way to go. Develop an argument complete with substantiating facts to support your position. We will get to both sides of the argument at the end of the book.

In short, this book is dedicated to the proposition that developing an informed base of knowledge constitutes an essential first step in reshaping the health care system as a social institution. The following chapters lay the groundwork. Given that this groundwork continues to shift, more attention will be necessary in the future to keep up with the terms of the debate. Personally, I find the topic fascinating. It is my hope that this book will stir an interest in you too and that it will provide a firm background that will challenge you to keep up with ongoing debates in the future. The more people are informed and interested, the more likely they will make better choices as we continue to rehab and reform this social institution over the twenty-first century.

2

Two Sociological Perspectives of the Health Care System

I know what you're thinking. Hillary Clinton and health care? Been there. Didn't do that!

No it's not 1994; it's 2004. And believe it or not, we have more problems today than we had back then. Issues like soaring health costs and millions of uninsured have to fix themselves.

Hillary Rodham Clinton
New York Times Magazine
April 18, 2004

Going without health insurance can have terrible consequences. The Institute of Medicine estimates that every year about 18,000 Americans die prematurely and unnecessarily because they do not have health care coverage. That is about two deaths per hour. While we meet here this morning, several of our fellow citizens are dying needlessly because they do not have health insurance.

Ronald F. Pollack
Executive director, Families USA
At the hearing on covering the uninsured before the
Democratic Policy Committee
United States Senate
January 6, 2004

If you found the basic sociological idea presented in the previous chapter to be reasonable — namely, that social institutions are constructed by members of a society as they go about the business of creating and then reshaping organizations to reflect a particular set of social values — then the discussion presented in this chapter should make sense to you as well. In the last chapter we focused on how such tangibles as structures and processes take shape. In this chapter we turn to something that is far less tangible than the construction of policies, programs, and organizations. We consider how people arrive at the *interpretations* they assign to the impact that those policies, programs, and organizations are having. Sociologists believe that people look at reality through interpretive frameworks. Why else would different people come up with varying interpretations when looking at the same reality? Sociologists are firmly convinced that such frameworks are acquired or learned. There is nothing innate or natural about it. If you get the idea that sociologists do not believe interpretations are entirely objective, you're right. When we refer to "the social construction of reality," we are referring to the process that explains how people interpret and come to understand what they see.

To illustrate, about forty or fifty years ago, society determined that wearing pierced earrings was fashionable. So, young women across the country began to have their ears pierced. Society was not nearly as sanguine when young men started piercing their ears but eventually got used to the idea. Since then society has been considering how to interpret pierced noses, lips, tongues, and other, less-visible body parts. Now the question, at least in some circles, is less a matter of whether piercing is acceptable but of how many earrings, nose rings, and so on one can accommodate at the same time without it being considered excessive. So do you think that government agencies in Washington, D.C., will soon be hiring people into high-level positions who have pierced lips? How would you feel about going to a doctor who was wearing a couple of tasteful little rings in his pierced eyebrow? What meaning do you attach to the decision to wear jewelry in pierced body parts—is it a statement? What kind of statement? Is it behavior that is equally acceptable for everyone? I am sure that you do not need to be told that people develop firm views about the answers to such questions. The fact that you may attach one meaning while other members of your family attach different meanings and that any one of you may change your respective opinions somewhere along the way means that piercing body parts does not come with a fully developed interpretation. Everyone who observes it, talks about it, and develops a position on how he or she feels about it is participating in the process of socially constructing the meaning of body piercing. This is what sociologists have in mind when they say that people construct the reality in which they live by assigning meanings to the behaviors of people around them.

We consider what sociologists think about the process of constructing reality at this point to explain how it is that people can look at reasonably objective data—the number of doctors' visits per person per year, for example—and argue whether the rate is appropriate, too high, or too low. Because there is often no objective answer, people turn to a belief system to interpret the facts. This helps people to define the situation, decide whether it is problematic, and offer solutions if they determine that the situation is sufficiently problematic. At this point, acknowledging the different frameworks for seeing and thinking about reality comes in. When sociologists look at the world, they do not all look at it in the same way, which is why sociology offers a choice of frameworks. As anyone who has taken an introductory course in sociology already knows, some sociological frameworks apply to interpersonal interactions between individuals whereas others are better suited to analyzing interactions among large groups of people. In this book most attention is given to programs, policies, and organizations, all of which involve large groups of people.

Accordingly, for purposes of this discussion, we will employ the two most encompassing lenses or frameworks—functionalist theory and conflict theory—to provide meaning to what we see when we look at the workings of the health care delivery system. If you want to quibble about it, neither qualifies as a true theory. They are perspectives or frameworks or schools of thought. They are not sufficiently worked out, testable, and "provable" to be theories. The reason the word *theory* comes into the discussion is that the conflict perspective has conventionally been called *conflict theory* even though most sociologists would agree that it is not really a theory. Some advocates of conflict theory are now calling it a "critical perspective" because it takes a critical stance and criticizes the performance of social institutions. Before you determine that the conflict theorists cannot make up their minds about their identity or that they are violating some truth-in-labeling norms, you should know that the functionalists are not entirely free of naming difficulties either. For many years the perspective was called *structural functionalism*, which is in fact a better label because it captures its essence more accurately. But that is a fairly cumbersome title. In any case, I use the functionalist and conflict theory labels for purposes of this discussion.

With this introduction to the sociological concepts addressed in this book, you now know what a social institution is and understand why sociologists say it has been socially constructed. In the remainder of this chapter, I explain the two theoretical perspectives just mentioned.

THE FUNCTIONALIST PERSPECTIVE

The essential difference between the two basic analytical perspectives sociology employs is in how those who espouse one or the other interpret what they see when they look at the same slice of the world. The functionalists look at society and see social order. For the most part, they see all the organizations, groups, and individuals working together to produce a reasonable degree of social equilibrium.

Functionalists argue that *structures* evolve and survive because they serve a social purpose, and by *structures*, I mean organizations, patterns of behavior, and groups; this is where the structuralism part of the original structural–functional label comes from. The social institution of the family comes to mind as an example. Society has a lot to say about family in general and marriage in particular—who should marry whom at what age, where they should live, how many children they should have, and so on (as you know, the question of whether gays should be allowed to marry has also been attracting a great deal of attention over the last couple of years). What is most interesting is that different societies have very firm ideas about the answers to these questions and that their answers are not the same. According to the functionalists, this is evidence that societies are actively creating and altering this social institution to meet what is a fundamental social need.

Aligning oneself with the functionalists' camp does not require that one agree with absolutely everything the functionalists have to say. There is always debate going on about the fine points that those outside of the camp often do not understand or care about. Belonging to this camp does, however, mean that one sees social institutions as structures that society is striving to shape in ways that will benefit society. Functionalists believe that society is capable of meeting its needs through the institutions it creates. They say that if an institution does not work well for a while, then other social institutions expand their activities to pick up those functions. As functionalists see it, society self-adjusts and self-regulates and provides us with a fair measure of stability and continuity. One might conclude that functionalists have a positive outlook. (The conflict theorists say they are being naïve.) They believe that society is not only capable of creating institutions that are beneficial to society but succeeds in doing so.

Functionalists argue that a better balance is achieved as social institutions drop some functions, add new ones, and make other adjustments. Social institutions do not fail; they change. The functionalists see the process of continuing adjustment as pretty remarkable considering that there is no CEO issuing orders and overseeing the process. They take pleasure in pointing out how society functions to bring various components into alignment to create social stability and continuity. After all, they say, most social institutions do work; they do meet society's needs. What is obvious to the functionalists is that, if this were not the case, then social institutions would change so that they could and would meet society's needs.

THE CONFLICT THEORY PERSPECTIVE

By contrast, when conflict theorists look at the same scene, they see disorder. More than that, they see the world divided into two segments—the "haves" and the "have-nots." What is there to "have"? One can have more money or more power or, likely, more of both. That does not settle it for the conflict theorists. As they see it, those who have more money and/or power are continually trying to protect their advantage, while those who have less money and/or power are trying to get more than they have. Battles between the two may or may not be overt and public.

To illustrate, when union members go out on strike to achieve better wages and working conditions, the terms of the conflict and the positions taken by the participants involved are obvious. While conflict theorists agree that anyone who is interested can watch the battle unfold and follow the negotiations, they argue that what transpires offstage is often far more important than what the public does see. This occurs because most people do not stop to consider the advantages that go with being in the position occupied by the haves.

What conflict theorists would say about the strike situation is that the issues being negotiated are really not as obvious as they might first appear. Most people know only what the media—television, newspapers, news magazines—report. The media do more than tell us what the issues are; they influence our perceptions through the selection of spokespersons for each side, the time devoted to each side, and so on. The conflict theorists would urge us to examine the details of such events more carefully than merely listening to the soundbites the media offer. They might point out that reporters seem readier to interview more representatives of management (the haves) than union members (the have-nots) and represent the former's views sympathetically. Therefore, it should not be surprising that the public ends up believing that the employer cannot afford to give the strikers what they are demanding. According to the conflict theorists, this explains why so many Americans are prepared to believe that workers who strike are fully aware that they are demanding unreasonable raises, that they knowingly risk bankrupting their employers, and that their demands are wild and unreasonable. When the organization closes down and moves its operations to a developing country where wages are much lower, the public does not blame management. In the end, Americans have no trouble believing that the strikers caused the displacement themselves.

According to the conflict theorists, how we perceive such events is determined by the behind-the-scenes influence of organizational owners and managers (other, like-minded haves). The owners and managers of large industrial organizations are likely to share the same worldviews as the owners of newspapers, television, and radio stations; and, even more important, the owners of all the other organizations who use those channels to advertise their products.

To clarify, conflict theorists do not traffic in conspiracy theories. They do not believe that the haves are doing anything as crude as getting together to plan their attack on the have-nots. Of course, the haves do get together at events that have nothing to do with planning such attacks, places such as the "club," board-of-trustees meetings of charitable organizations or charity balls, and parties thrown by people who have earned a great deal of money and are eager to mix with the more established haves. Conflict theorists would not say that there is a conspiracy brewing here; what they would say is that it is interesting that the views of the rich and powerful just happen to be the views that are articulated most clearly in the media and that most of us end up accepting those views as truth.

The conflict theorists would also point out that the haves help their cause by making every effort to convince the have-nots that they, too, can join the forces of the rich and famous if they work at it. After all, this is a free country and any-one can do it. At this point, they may offer examples of the rise from ordinary beginnings to riches achieved by a few easily recognizable individuals. The position advocated by the haves is that society must, of course, ensure that the right incentives exist, such as being able to keep more of what people earn, which will happen if society quits giving lazy, dishonest, drug-abusing people a free ride.

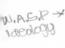

As the conflict theorists see it, this line of thought actually has the effect of keeping everyone in his or her respective place. The haves get to keep a far greater amount of income than those who earn less. The conflict theorists point out that very few people do make it to the top—that is, the top of the income scale. However, promoting such a point of view helps to keep the system intact, meaning that the haves continue to have much more money and power than the average American. Put into sociological terms, the effect is highly conservatizing. The conflict theorists are not terribly hopeful that Americans will suddenly see things differently in the future. One might conclude that the conflict theorists are far more pessimistic than the functionalists with regard to the role played by social institutions and the likelihood that any changes that occur in the structure of social institutions will be beneficial to anyone but the haves.

HEALTH CARE AS A SOCIAL INSTITUTION

Now that you see where those who align themselves with these two basic sociological perspectives are coming from, we now look at the health care delivery system through the lenses provided by each group.

The Functionalists

According to the functionalists, the health care system evolved to address the widely shared need for health care. The policies, programs, and organizations that make up this social institution were created to accomplish particular objectives, which are the *manifest functions*. Manifest functions are the goals that the social institution proclaims in its public statements about its activities. Thus, as the functionalists see it, the health care system is trying its best to

- Keep people healthy so that they can fulfill their normal responsibilities — namely, going to work or attending school, which are essential for ensuring social continuity and stability
- Educate and promote healthy behavior and issue warnings regarding those that are unhealthy — whether these are voluntary, such as smoking, or involuntary, such as exposure to carcinogenic airborne pollutants
- Increase scientific knowledge and capability to intervene in cases of serious illness by improving diagnostic tools, surgical techniques, medications, and so on
- Offer comfort and alleviate pain in the case of patients with illnesses for which medicine has no cure

Functionalists recognize that there are also some things that social institutions do that they were not officially designed to do. Functionalists call these the *latent functions*. The latent functions performed by the health care system include

- Providing jobs for a large number of people
- Providing selected individuals, usually doctors, the opportunity to develop impressive reputations based on forging ahead into new medical/scientific frontiers
- Building a hospital that stands as a "repository of community values" — that is, it symbolizes the community's identity, its religious, ethnic, and other special and identifiable characteristic, such as a connection to a university[1]
- Using the hospital, once it exists, to bring members of the community together to set up activities that would benefit the community as whole, such as training programs, patient education programs, programs to help the poor, and so on

The Conflict Theorists

We now turn to the conflict theory perspective on the role performed by the health care delivery system as a social institution. The conflict theorists do not separate the functions performed by social institutions into manifest and latent. Conflict theorists believe that saying something is a manifest function simply means that one has "bought into" the propaganda put forth by the haves.

Conflict theorists do not assign priorities or differentiate in any way among the purposes they see being fulfilled by any social institution, nor do they group themselves into different categories based on variations in interest. There are, however, two rather distinct factions of conflict theorists actively engaged in critiquing health care delivery system arrangements at present. It is not that they disagree with each other but that their observations are addressed to different levels of behavior. I distinguish between conflict theorists who are concerned with *microlevel interactions* and those who focus on *macrolevel interactions*.

When sociologists talk about microlevel interactions, they mean the kinds of exchanges—that is, talk and behavior—that go on between two people or, at most, a small number people. Conflict theorists who focus on the microlevel say that this social institution has the following characteristics:

- It has established norms that reinforce the dominance of physicians over patients; this is especially apparent when the physician is a male and the patient is a female or when the physician is white and the patient is a member of an ethnic or racial minority group.
- It has created organizational structures—that is, hospitals, licensure arrangements, and so forth—that perpetuate the dominance and power of physicians over other health care workers.
- It denies the legitimacy of patients' experiences by ignoring patients' complaints for which doctors have no objective measures; this is a criticism of the medical model explanation for disease, which I explain next.

Most medical sociologists, both functionalists and conflict theorists, tend to be critical of the "medical model" explanation of illness, but as might be expected, those who are more firmly attached to the conflict theory camp are more critical. What sociologists say is that by controlling what constitutes "disease," doctors are actively engaged in the social control of behavior. They have set themselves up as the arbiters of what is a legitimate illness versus an illegitimate one. (We will return to this issue in chapter 5 when we consider it from the doctors' perspective.) To illustrate, alcoholics would like us to believe that their addiction to alcohol is biologically based. Doctors say that the evidence substantiating that claim is more complicated. There may be a genetic predisposition, but that does not mean that everyone with this trait will become an alcoholic. The question of whether it is biological affects how society looks at persons who have this problem. If alcoholism is biological, then

•

it is a disease and people cannot be blamed for it. If, however, the biological basis is less clear-cut, then society presumes there is a large measure of moral failure involved. In that case, it is logical to conclude that people can choose to stop drinking and causing all the problems that drunkenness produces and that those who do not stop are simply morally weak, so society should not be forgiving.

In short, the medical model is what is responsible for doctors deciding to regard certain types of problems, such as alcoholism, as falling outside the realm of medical care. Of course, once the drinking produces liver disease, doctors can and do identify it as a biologically based medical problem and use all the resources at their disposal to treat that medical condition.

Conflict theorists criticize doctors not only for ignoring some of the problems patients bring to them but also for claiming too much that is characteristically human as legitimate territory for medical intervention. In fact, this is the more common criticism. Sociologists call this *medicalization*. Conflict theorists say that doctors have taken it upon themselves to define a whole range of features of normal life as appropriate for medical intervention. They prescribe medications to help people sleep, help them stay alert, increase their energy level, help them build bigger muscles, and so on. Plastic surgeons set standards of beauty when they reshape patients' bodies, do nose jobs, face lifts, tummy tucks, provide breast implants, and so on. Normal variations are being named and treated as if they were diseases. For example, PMS (premenstrual stress syndrome) and menopause are no longer considered to be a normal part of life but syndromes that require medication. All this grows out of the "medical model" doctors use to separate what they are willing to treat from what they have no interest in treating. At the heart of this criticism is the idea that doctors make these determinations to advance their own interests rather than patients' interests. It reinforces their power and control over others.

The other faction of conflict theorists, who focus on macrolevel interactions (rather than microlevel, interpersonal interactions), do not consider the impact on individuals to be the most important issue to be addressed. They are more interested in the impact that this social institution, in contrast to individual doctors, has on society as a whole. This faction looks at reality and sees large categories of people being affected by the structures and processes that operate within the health care system. As they see it, the whole health care system is highly conservatizing in the way it operates, as illustrated by its characteristics:

• It replicates the social structure by providing better health care services for the haves than for the have-nots.

- By connecting health insurance to employment, it justifies giving poorer care to the have-nots by suggesting that they do not need or deserve care that is as good as the level of care available to the haves. Thus, it not only replicates the social structure but reinforces the effects of the circumstances that people are born into.
- It replicates the social hierarchy in its division of labor, which results in women and minorities having lower status and lower-paying jobs.

Sometimes the arguments within each of the two theoretical camps break out to attract wider interest—admittedly, wider interest here means that among a wider spectrum of sociologists. Thus, we find that a few conflict theorists have made it clear that they completely disagree with fellow conflict theorists who criticize doctors for the degree of dominance they display. This faction of conflict theorists argues that the medical dominance that some sociologists have criticized so thoroughly is puffery and self-delusion on the part of doctors. They say that the reality is that doctors do not have nearly as much power as we have been led to believe. According to this group of conflict theorists, doctors are merely serving the purposes of a really powerful class of people—the capitalists who benefit from the profits that the U.S. health care delivery arrangements produce for them.

Consider the evidence they offer. They say that Americans have a much higher surgical rate than people in other countries do because major corporations have had more to gain from supporting this form of treatment than the kind of medical care that is provided by doctors who do not perform surgery. They blame the medical–industrial complex. (It is worth noting that a 1971 issue of *Fortune* magazine advised its readers to invest in the "medical–industrial complex," so the label cannot be considered a fantasy concocted by a radical faction of conflict theorists.) The medical–industrial complex requires a steady demand for new products—sophisticated monitoring machines, vast quantities of hospital supplies (all of which are now disposable), ever-improving diagnostic equipment, and so on. Because such products are used in hospitals rather than doctors' offices, the medical–industrial complex was interested in advancing a surgical approach to resolving health problems whenever possible. The capitalists have allowed doctors who are interested in doing so to take the credit, bask in the glory, and generally become insufferable in their interactions with patients and other health care workers as long as doing so did not interfere with the capitalists' agenda of making more money.

In the meantime, doctors who practice medicine (versus surgery), taking long medical histories and advising their patients to change their lifestyles, had not been receiving nearly as much support from the capitalists, because they used few saleable products in the process. From the capitalists' perspective, there was little reason to support doctors working in their own offices as opposed to hospitals because they were offering little profit-making potential.

But, things change, and capitalists are the first to admit that they are very flexible when it comes to promising investments. It seems that all the effort that went into supporting surgical advances has had the somewhat unanticipated effect of developing new forms of surgery that are less invasive (smaller incisions are made with the increased use of lasers). This has reduced the number of days patients need to stay in the hospital; it has put many hospitals out of business; and it has reduced the need for so many surgeons. Physicians (who are not surgeons) are suddenly attracting the interest of capitalists.

There are a number of related trends that are contributing to this revision in capitalist thinking. Because capitalists are sensitive to shifts in market conditions, they recognize that the United States, like most industrialized countries, is an aging society. That means more people are living longer, but the chances are good that they are living with an increasing number of chronic diseases and are taking multiple medications. Accordingly, the capitalists have been investing in the pharmaceutical industry, which is one of the most profitable industries in the country (a trend we will discuss in more detail later). The conflict theorists see this as evidence that doctors who prescribe medicine as opposed to doing surgery are gaining greater influence, not because of anything they have done, but because it is in the interests of capitalists to have this happen. In short, according to conflict theorists, doctors do not now have, nor have they ever had, total control over the health care system.

THE CHAPTERS TO FOLLOW

So who is right? Is the health care delivery system basically functional and merely going through some minor adjustments to better meet society's needs? That is, of course, the functionalists' position. Or, are the changes that are occurring happening without much input from the majority of Americans but a great deal of input from the "haves"? The latter sums up the conflict theory perspective. Sociology, as a discipline, is not organized to offer a single answer; each person must decide for himself or herself.

There is no question that the conflict theory perspective has been winning out over the functionalist perspective among medical sociologists for quite some time. As a result, the conflict theory perspective will probably look stronger than the functionalist perspective in the following chapters. Of course, it is not only sociologists who see a lot to criticize when they look at current health care delivery arrangements.

Another reason that the conflict position appears stronger is that the functionalists are not as vocal as the conflict theorists, so it is not always easy to represent their thoughts on many of these issues. Functionalists were far more vocal in the past. It is also true that the characteristics of the health care delivery system that the functionalists said were working so well then have changed. What they said was especially functional in the past no longer exists. Those arrangements have been replaced by new arrangements, with a central feature being the commitment to a corporate, business approach to operating health care organizations. It is unlikely that functionalists intended to support the way things have evolved. However, committing oneself to a functionalist view of the world does carry with it the need to say that current arrangements are working well or that society would make the appropriate adjustments. Accordingly, those who espouse the functionalist perspective must now logically favor such mechanisms as competition, marketing, and corporate health-sector organizational expansion or be prepared to argue that current arrangements are not "functional." The current state of the health care delivery system is not one many functionalists are eager to defend in the face of increasing public dissatisfaction and the biting criticism of colleagues who are conflict theorists. In the last chapter of the book, we will return to the question of what this says about the relationship between the two theoretical perspectives.

The observation that the conflict theorists are more vocal than the functionalists should not surprise too many people. Just look at the stories that are reported by the news media. As everybody knows, the sensational stuff gets the most attention. The "good guy" stories are reported in specially dedicated segments, as rarities to be marveled at. It is difficult to find people saying positive things about the way most things operate, a fact not limited to the health care system. When people do say positive things, they often do so in response to more specific criticisms. That tends to make such people sound defensive at best and, at worst, intent on distorting what we have already become convinced is terrible but true. As I repeat more than once in the pages to follow, it is not easy to sort out the facts.

Numerous problems plaguing the health sector have been identified in recent years. Which problems are the most pressing is, of course, in the eye of the beholder. That is to say, people have come up with very different "definitions of the situation," which explains why there are so many different solutions being promoted and why those solutions are so different from one another. And that, in a nutshell, is why improving social institutions turns out to be so problematic.

What I propose to do in the body of the book is to identify in greater detail the structures and processes that make up the health care delivery system as a social institution. I apply both theoretical lenses discussed in this chapter to look at some of those processes and structures. Although all parts of the health care system are linked, we will examine various parts separately.

NOTE

1. Rosemary Stevens, *In Sickness and in Wealth* (New York: Basic Books, 1989).

3

What Do We Think of the U.S. Health Care System?

Given the probable long-term nature of international tensions and the terrorist threat, the uninsured and the health care issue in general are not likely to attain the same visibility in the near future that they had in the early 1990s. . . . On the other hand, dissatisfaction has been rising recently and the public remains concerned about the sluggish condition of the economy, often a harbinger of interest in the uninsured.

Robert J. Blendon, John M. Benson, and Catherine M. DesRoches
Health Affairs, web exclusive
August 27, 2003

18% of the physicians and 24% of the public said the [medical] error had caused serious consequences such as death, long-term disability or severe pain. . . . Despite these numbers, only 5% of the doctors and 6% of the public saw reducing medical errors as a top health concern. Physicians listed medical liability insurance costs and lawsuits as their top concern (29%), with health care costs close behind (27%). The public picked health care costs (38%) and prescription drug costs (31%) as its top concerns.

Andis Robeznieks
American Medical News
January 13, 2003

If you ask Americans what they think about our health care system, you are likely to hear a long list of things that are wrong with it. However, the same Americans are also likely to end by saying that, in spite of all that, this is still the best system in the world. Sociologists would say this is an example of *ethnocentrism*. It means that we think "ours is best" simply because it is "ours" (whatever "ours" refers to at the moment). When ethnocentrism kicks in, people resent being asked to explain why they prefer what they prefer; nor are they pleased to be asked to provide some evidence to show that it—whatever "it" is—is in fact better in some way. In actuality, no matter how much effort one is willing to put into being "health-care-delivery-system-centric," saying that our health system is the best just does not stand up in the face of reality no matter how much we would like it to.

Consider the most basic indicators. First, Americans do not live as long as people in many other developed and developing countries. According to the U.S. Department of Health and Human Services, males live longer in twenty-four of thirty-seven of those countries and women live longer in twenty-one.[1] Second, our infant mortality rate (death of babies under one year of age) is higher than it is in twenty-eight out of the same thirty-seven countries.[2] This is important because infant mortality is considered the most sensitive measure of the health of a society—namely, because babies are the most vulnerable. Third, for this we pay more than anyone else in the world.

So what makes our system the best? It's our technology, right? We have the best medical technology in the world, and we have lots of it. After all, people from all over the world come here to have operations. So, why isn't all that technology doing much for our life expectancy? Because people smoke, drink, eat the wrong things, don't exercise? Anyone who travels to other countries cannot help but notice that people in other countries smoke a lot more, drink more, eat rich foods, do not exercise, and still live a lot longer. Look at the French!

Maybe it's because there is something wrong with the way our health system is organized. When pressed, the defenders of our health care system are willing to acknowledge that everyone does not necessarily benefit from our technology. Not because it isn't there, they point out, but because people are not making the effort to take advantage of what is readily available. Almost everyone involved in studying the health care delivery system would say, "That's stretching it." The defenders generally go on to say that our technology is the best and available to everyone; public hospitals have it available and will provide it for free to those who really cannot pay for it; and if people don't use it, there is nothing you can do to make them use it. There are a couple of assumptions in these statements that deserve further exploration. For one, the statements suggest that the level of technology in other countries is not as advanced. That is not true in the case of the major industrialized European countries and Japan. They have the same kind of technology, only not as much as we have. (We will look at systems in other countries in chapter 10.) The second built-in assumption is that more technology is always better. After all you can get a CT (computerized axial tomography) scan on every corner in this country and that's great—right? In actuality, health policy makers in the United States and other countries discovered a couple of decades ago that the doctors and technicians who perform various "high-tech" procedures and tests must do a certain number of them on a regular basis to maintain a high level of proficiency. Having many machines simply means that the people operating them, or worse yet interpreting the results, are not experienced enough to do a good job—to recognize aberrations, to interpret the significance of subtle differences, and so on. Not only is that hard to hear, but it strikes at the heart of the claim that more technology is always good.

Where does that leave us in evaluating our health care system? For years, a sizable proportion of Americans said that our health care system is in a state of crisis. How can we say that we have the best health care system in the world one minute and say that the system is in crisis the next minute? In part, different people say these things. Whatever the explanation for such inconsistency, it will be helpful to look at the evidence.

EXACTLY WHAT HAVE WE BEEN SAYING ABOUT THE SYSTEM?

So how do we really know how satisfied or dissatisfied Americans are with current health care delivery system arrangements? Is it possible that all the talk about problems related to our health care arrangements is just another example of media hype or is of concern only to the elderly who rely on Medicare, or maybe it was and still is of greater interest to academics than anyone else? Yet, it is hard to miss the number of news reports, magazine stories, and television specials that focus on some aspect of health, health care services, and health care costs. As we all know, such reports would not be so common unless the media watchers had established that those stories would attract large audiences.

On this point it is interesting to note that health care executives have been known to complain that public opinion is shaped by the news media, which have been at certain times unduly critical of how health care organizations treat patients.[3] An analysis of the content of news publications and network news broadcasts between 1990 and 1997 indicates that the stories did become more critical over that time.[4] Reporters did dramatize single incidents and end up identifying insurance companies and the health care organizations they sponsor as the "villains" in their stories.

There is, of course, no way to know how much of the dissatisfaction with the health care system expressed by Americans can be attributed to the negative reports found in the media. What we can do is continue to ask the public what it thinks about the workings of the health care system on a regular basis to trace shifts in public opinion, even if we cannot always be sure why those shifts are occurring. This idea suggests that we should be looking at the results of opinion polls, especially polls conducted by well-known survey research organizations and summarized by respected scholars. Most of the public opinion material presented here is based on surveys conducted by a team of researchers associated with the School of Public Health at Harvard University. We begin by examining what these researchers can tell us about the attitudes regarding health care arrangements expressed by Americans over the last half of the twentieth century.

PUBLIC OPINION SURVEYS OVER THE LAST HALF-CENTURY

The scholars I just mentioned examined about one hundred public opinion surveys linked to the four periods during which health care reform was seriously debated in this country:

- Late 1940s, the Truman era
- 1961–1965, the Kennedy/Johnson era
- 1971–1974, the Nixon era
- 1993–1994, the Clinton era[5]

Public interest and support were initially high during each of these periods. However, major pieces of legislation were enacted during the Kennedy/Johnson and Nixon eras but not the Truman and Clinton eras. During the first of the four periods, the Truman years, 82 percent of the public favored doing something to help people pay for health care, with 68 percent agreeing that using social security as the basis for enacting a universal health care plan was a good idea. Yet, the reform legislation being discussed at that time failed to pass. During the subsequent period examined, the Kennedy/Johnson era, 75 percent of Americans favored a plan to provide medical care for seniors. That brought the Medicare program into existence. During the third period, the Nixon era, no comparable survey was conducted, so there is no record documenting the prevailing level of public support for legislative reform. What we do know is that a major piece of health legislation, creating health maintenance organizations, was enacted during the Nixon presidency. A review of opinion polls conducted during the fourth period, the early years of the Clinton era, indicates that 66 percent of Americans were prepared to support legislation creating a tax-funded national health insurance plan. However, the Clinton reform proposal did not make it through the legislative process.

The researchers went on to examine how the four periods differed, in an effort to understand what accounts for either the success or failure of reform proposals. One distinguishing characteristic across the four periods was the rate at which public support fell once the health care plans began to take shape. Decline in support was more rapid during the Truman and Clinton administrations.

The researchers' second conclusion is more consequential. They identified two factors that turned out to be critical in determining whether reforms are actually enacted—namely, the level of trust in government and the feelings about federal taxes. While there is strong evidence that trust in government has been steadily eroding since the 1950s, they point out that the level of distrust in government was especially high during the Clinton era. We also know that federal taxes have never been popular in this country but that taxation was considerably *less unpopular* during the 1960s—that is, during the Kennedy/Johnson era. Indeed, the public was willing to pay higher taxes to support health care for the elderly. To sum up, Americans have consistently expressed dissatisfaction with the health care system in this country. And they have been just as consistent in their reluctance to support solutions that depend on either greater government involvement or increased taxes.

This does not mean that Americans think the country spends too much on health care. In fact, at no point over the last fifty years of the twentieth century have more than 9 percent of Americans said that the country spends too much. What displeases Americans is how much they must spend out of their own pockets, not how much the country as a whole spends. Curiously, Americans have not been particularly interested in examining the connection between these two forms of expenditure. How much the country spends on health care is calculated as a percentage of the gross domestic product (GDP). We should discuss this concept in a little more detail.

GDP AND WHAT WE PAY FOR OUR HEALTH CARE

The GDP is a measure of the total of goods and services produced by everyone in the country. That is certainly a straightforward definition until you start thinking about what it means. It becomes daunting if you conceptualize it as a pie chart and understand that *all* goods and services produced or purchased by anyone and everyone in the country must fit into the pie—cell phones, cars, bridges, bombs, dental care, computers, the space program, food stamps, houses, police protection, rock concerts, and so forth. The slice of this pie that goes to health care products and services has been getting bigger over the years. Throughout the 1990s, it hovered around 14 percent. As of 2003, it jumped to 15.3 percent. Think of that as about fifteen cents out of every dollar spent on anything and everything in this country. Is that too much, too little, about right? How do we know? Experts, especially economists, have lots of opinions on how you might evaluate that figure.

One way to evaluate it is to compare how much we spend with how much people in other countries spend. We will do that shortly and go on to compare those results to how satisfied people in other countries say they are with their respective health care arrangements.

SATISFACTION IN THE UNITED STATES COMPARED TO OTHER COUNTRIES

The expense involved in conducting international surveys prevents pollsters from conducting them on a regular basis, but those that have been carried out are especially informative. Particularly striking are the results of a comparative international study reported in 1990. A random sample of people in ten advanced industrialized countries was asked to evaluate their health care arrangements. Table 3.1 shows the proportion of people who agreed with the following statement: "On the whole, the health care system works pretty well, and only minor changes are necessary to make it work better." The alternative options were "There are some good things in our health system, but fundamental changes are needed to make it work better" and "Our health care system has so much wrong with it that we need to completely rebuild it." Those who selected the first answer are identified here as *highly satisfied,* as opposed to *moderately satisfied* or *dissatisfied,* with the country's health care arrangements. Looking at the column, you can see that the countries are arrayed from highest to lowest in the level of satisfaction they registered.

The data presented in table 3.1 tell us that Americans, in comparison to people in all those other highly industrialized countries, were at the low end of the spectrum on satisfaction in 1990. Comparing the first two columns, on satisfaction and GDP, reveals something of a pattern. While the correlation is not perfect, it seems that the more a country spent on health care, the more satisfied the people were with their health care arrangements. The United States was the major exception. In short, we were spending the most on health care, and we were the least satisfied. Comparing national expenditures to the last two columns on life expectancy is also revealing. Don't you find it interesting to see that spending more on health care is not necessarily consistent with longer life expectancy? All in all, the table seems to indicate that the United States was not spending its health care dollars very effectively. Although there is no update available on the satisfaction portion of this table, we

Table 3.1. Percentage of People Satisfied with Health Care, Percentage of Gross Domestic Product (GDP) Spent on Health Care, and Life Expectancy (1990)

	Satisfaction %	GDP: Health care %	Life expectancy	
			M	F
Canada	56	9.4	74.4	81.0
Netherlands	47	8.2	74.1	80.4
France	41	8.9	73.5	82.0
W. Germany	41	8.3	72.7	79.2
Australia	34	8.2	73.2	76.4
Sweden	32	8.6	74.9	80.6
Japan	29	6.6	76.4	82.8
England/Wales	27	6.2	73.5	79.0
Italy	12	8.1	73.7	78.5
U.S.	10	12.6	72.0	78.9

Sources: Robert Blendon, Robert Leitman, Ian Morrison, and Karen Donelan, "Satisfaction with Health Systems in Ten Nations," *Health Affairs* (Summer 1990): 185–92; "Total Health Expenditures as a Percentage of Gross Domestic Product per Capita Health Expenditures in Dollars: Selected Countries and Years 1960–93," *Health United States*, 1995 (Washington, D.C.: U.S. Department of Health and Human Services, Public Health Service, 1996), table 115; "Life Expectancy at Birth and at 65 Years of Age, according to Sex: Selected Countries, 1987–1992," *Health United States*, 1995 (Washington, D.C.: U.S. Department of Health and Human Services, Public Health Service, 1996), table 28.

do know that we are still spending more than all those other countries and that we are still not living as long as those countries' citizens.

PUBLIC OPINION OVER THE LAST DECADE OF THE TWENTIETH CENTURY AND BEYOND

The results of this international satisfaction survey indicate that the public was highly dissatisfied with prevailing health care arrangements during the early 1990s. This is the era during which the Clinton presidential campaign promised and ultimately delivered a health care reform agenda. Based on the analysis presented earlier on factors that cause reform plans to die away, we know that the Clinton reform effort failed because the plan could not overcome the two most basic obstacles that confront health care reform efforts—Americans' distrust of government and their objection to higher taxes. Institutional resistance to change presented another obstacle. Once the structures created by social institutions come into existence—in this case the health policies, programs, and organizations—they resist change. Social institutions do change, but they change slowly. The Clinton healthcare reform effort was pretty much designed to reorganize the whole health care system. That turned out to be far too radical an approach for addressing dissatisfaction.

Another obstacle to the Clinton reform effort stems from the difficulty Americans have agreeing on what health care delivery problems need to be fixed, let alone how to fix them. (You can see how the "definition of the prob-lem" is a reflection of the "social construction of reality.") Americans were still not sure whether they wanted everyone in the country insured or just those who "deserved" it. However, that was then. A shift in attitude occurred by the end of decade. By the first few years of the twenty-first century, Amer-icans registered far more willingness to support insurance for everyone.[6]

To understand the shift in attitude regarding who should be insured in this country, it is important to review the changes in health care arrangements that occurred during the health reform discussions of the early Clinton years. In-terested parties did not stand around waiting to see what would happen. They actively prepared for the possibility that the plan would be enacted. The in-surance industry in particular took steps to solidify its position so that it could fight off government incursion into its affairs. As a result, the insurance in-dustry was well positioned when the Clinton plan failed. Not surprisingly, health insurance costs continued to increase in the wake of the failed plan. Employers responded by reducing the insurance coverage options they were offering to their employees, which the insurance industry did not mind since employers were still buying health insurance. Public dissatisfaction about health care arrangements did not increase as much as might be expected in re-sponse to the reduction in insurance options, because the economy was boom-ing and unemployment rates were low. Americans were not nearly as worried about health insurance over the second half of the decade as they were at the beginning of the Clinton presidency, when the economy was much weaker.[7]

However, the public did begin to worry that the cutbacks on coverage might affect the quality of care they were receiving, a topic about which Americans did not register much concern in the past. A 1997 survey found that three-quarters of people in the country thought there were "serious prob-lems with the quality of health care." About 70 percent said that hospitals were cutting costs to save money and that insurance companies were not only primarily interested in saving money but did not care if peoples' health was being compromised.[8]

SATISFACTION RATES IN THE WAKE OF SEPTEMBER 11

A May 2001 public opinion survey on national priorities found Americans most concerned about health care, jobs, education, and the economy.[9] As we all know, national priorities shifted dramatically just a few months later in re-sponse to the events of September 11. War, defense, and terrorism moved to the top of the list of national concerns, leaving health care tied with education for fourth place. This shift in priorities was clearly documented in a survey conducted the following year by the Harvard team of researchers, just before the 2002 congressional elections.[10] The researchers wanted to determine where concern about health care issues stood compared to the other issues being discussed during the election season. They found that of those who said they were likely to vote, only 20 percent agreed with the following statement: "The American health care system has so much wrong with it that it needs to be completely rebuilt." Of those who were not likely to vote, 32 percent agreed. The researchers noted that there was good reason to consider this a significant difference.

What do you make of the fact that the people who are most unhappy about the situation are also the ones who do not plan to use their vote to try to change things? A number of observers have noted that a growing segment of society has been feeling powerless to change things and is giving up hope that their vote will make a difference This has serious social implications. It indicates a lack of confidence in both the health care system and the political system as social institutions. If people do not feel that they have much influence over how social institutions are constructed, then they are likely to feel that the institutions' rules do not apply to them, which in turn threatens the democratic basis of our society and ultimately risks the breakdown of social norms and understandings. The lack of confidence in and connection to the processes through which our social institutions evolve explains everything from why people run red lights to why those who are in a position to engage in corporate fraud do so. The findings on voting behavior are being interpreted by some as evidence that it is the poor and downtrodden—that is, the have-nots—who are increasingly feeling this way, which is, of course, not surprising. What is surprising is the recent discovery that such feelings contribute to their poor health to a greater extent than anyone had realized.[11] By not voting they are, in essence, helping to effect a "self-fulfilling prophecy."

A closer look at the views of those who said they were likely to vote provides us with specific information. Table 3.2 indicates which political party prospective voters believed was better equipped to deal with the public's main concerns.

According to the researchers who carried out this study, the results indicate that Americans may have been dissatisfied with the availability and affordability of health care but that health care ended up playing a modest role in determining the outcome of the 2002 congressional elections. For purposes of this discussion, it is the difference in presumed competence in table 3.2 by political party affiliation that we should attend to closely. In case you did not notice, the lists by party affiliation go in opposite directions, which can be interpreted to mean that our political leaders do not see the problems on this list from the same perspective. Not being able to agree on a list of national priorities

Table 3.2. Percentage of Prospective Voters Who Perceive One Political Party as Being Better Able to Handle Various Issues

	Republicans	Democrats
War on terrorism	61%	26%
Iraq and Saddam Hussein	58	31
Economy and jobs	48	43
Education	45	44
Health care	39	50
Social security	39	51
Prescription drugs for elderly	36	53

Source: Robert Blendon, Mollyann Brodie, Drew Altman, John Benson, Stephen Pelletier, and Marcus Rosenbaum, "Where Was Health Care in the 2002 Election?" *Health Affairs* web exclusive (December 11, 2002): 426–32.

prevents society from reaching a consensus regarding how to distribute the resources required to address the problems connected to these issues. There is no reason to expect this situation to change anytime soon. Providing further support for such an interpretation is an analysis of public opinion surveys conducted in 2003 that were designed to assess Americans' views on enacting legislation to provide health insurance for those who are uninsured. The survey results indicate that increasing numbers of Americans agreed that something should be done to help the uninsured; however, there was no consensus on any one approach for doing so.[12] Let us review a few of the report's highlights:

- In sum, 74 percent of Americans said that it was "extremely/very important to pass a law in the next year to provide health insurance for most uninsured Americans" in 2003.
- By party, 85 percent of Democrats agreed with the aforementioned statement, in contrast to 64 percent of Republicans. The pollsters noted that a difference of this magnitude, 21 percent, is substantial.
- When presented with a question asking if the only way to ensure that everyone gets health care is to raise taxes, 43 percent of Americans agreed, which breaks down into 53 percent of Democrats and 35 percent of Republicans.
- More revealing is the difference in attitude regarding the tax cut passed that year; 50 percent of Americans said it was a good thing, but that breaks down into 38 percent of Democrats, compared to an overwhelming majority of Republicans at 70 percent

These findings bring us back to the analysis of the fate of health reform proposals over the last half-century. You cannot help but conclude that Americans may not agree on many things, but enough Americans dislike taxes and distrust government to make designing health care arrangements to provide health insurance for everyone in the country a major hurdle. That is not to say that policy makers are about to give up on trying to alter our health care arrangements. It is to say that major reform is unlikely. Given the fact that the limited legislative reforms that have been enacted in recent years have neither helped to extend insurance coverage to large numbers of people nor succeeded in curtailing rising costs, we should expect Americans to continue reporting that they are dissatisfied with this country's health care arrangements. Although we can expect those sentiments to generate new health reform proposals, there is no reason to expect any of the new proposals to attract the support of the majority of Americans. It is hard to imagine what conditions would cause Americans to begin investing greater trust in the government or cause us to be more willing to see our taxes increased to support a new health reform plan.

WHERE DO WE GO FROM HERE?

Just in case you are beginning to think that there are no aspects of the health care system that we as a society can agree on, you will be pleased to hear that health policy makers and most other interested observers do agree on the three guiding principles that have shaped the structure of our health care arrangements for at least the last five decades. They are not formally documented and written down anywhere for good reason — that is, we do not have "a system." Nevertheless, here they are:

1. Attain the highest quality care.
2. Ensure access to care.
3. Contain costs.

Great goals, right? Unfortunately, that is where things fall apart because these three objectives are impossible to define concretely and are even more difficult to measure. What does *quality* mean? Who should define it? Doctors, patients, or some group of experts authorized (by whom?) to monitor quality? How much access? Access for everyone? Assurance that we can have all the health care services we want? Or that we can pay for? How do we measure cost containment? Do we want costs to drop or just not go up so fast? Are we prepared to cut anything? We will review the literature that addresses such questions in the following chapters.

At this point, what we can say for certain is that this social institution, like all the others, is the product of human effort. And as is always the case, the process of constructing it and rehabilitating it has not been particularly neat and orderly. We also know that the rehabilitation process is not about to stop, even though a growing number of observers have been saying that what we have collectively created is poorly organized, convoluted, and difficult to understand — in short, a mess.

In the chapters that follow I discuss the evolution of our unsystematic health care system using the following not particularly discrete topics: the people who are involved in delivering those services; the structures through which we receive health care services; and how we pay for the health care services we receive.

NOTES

1. "Life Expectancy at Birth and at 65 Years of Age, according to Sex: Selected Countries, Selected Years 1980–1998," *Health United States, 2003* (Washington, D.C.: U.S. Department of Health and Human Services, Public Health Service, 2003), table 26.

2. "Infant Mortality Rates and International Rankings: Selected Countries, Selected Years 1960–1999," *Health United States, 2003* (Washington, D.C.: U.S. Department of Health and Human Services, Public Health Service, 2003), table 25.

3. Karen Ignani, "Covering a Breaking Revolution: The Media and Managed Care," *Health Affairs* 17 (January/February 1998): 26–34.

4. Mollyann Brodie, Lee Ann Brady, and Drew Altman, "Media Coverage of Managed Care: Is There a Negative Bias?" *Health Affairs* 17 (January/February 1998): 9–25.

5. Robert Blendon and John Benson, "Americans' Views on Health Policy: A Fifty-Year Historical Perspective," *Health Affairs* 20 (March/April, 2001): 33–46.

6. Robert Blendon, John Benson, and Catherine DesRoches, "Americans' Views of the Uninsured: An Era for Hybrid Proposals," *Health Affairs* web exclusive (August 27, 2003): 405–14.

7. Robert Blendon, Tracey Stelzer Hyams, and John Benson, "Bridging the Gap between Expert and Public Views on Health Care Reform," *Journal of the American Medical Association* 269 (May 19, 1993): 2573–78.

8. Robert Brook, Caren Kamberg, and Elizabeth McGlynn, "Health System Reform and Quality," *Journal of the American Medical Association* 276 (August 14, 1996): 476–80.

9. Robert Blendon, Catherine DesRoches, John Young, and Kimberly Scoles, "The Impact of Terrorism and the Recession on Americans' Health Priorities," *Health Affairs* web exclusive (January 16, 2002): 420–25.

10. Robert Blendon, Mollyann Brodie, Drew Altman, John Benson, Stephen Pelletier, and Marcus Rosenbaum, "Where Was Health Care in the 2002 Election?" *Health Affairs* web exclusive (December 11, 2002): 426–32.

11. Tony Blakely, Bruce Kennedy, and Ichiro Kawachi, "Socioeconomic Inequality in Voting Participation and Self-Rated Health," *American Journal of Public Health* 91 (January 2001): 99–104; Ichiro Kawachi, Bruce Kennedy, and Richard Wilkinson, *The Population Health Reader*, vol. 1 (New York: New Press, 1999).

12. Blendon, Benson, and DesRoches, "Americans' Views of the Uninsured."

4

Hospitals and Other Health Care Organizations

Press Release: American Hospital Association charged as a defendant in class action lawsuits brought by uninsured patients against nonprofit hospital system and hospitals. . . . Among other things, the AHA encourages its co-defendant nonprofit hospital systems and hospitals to perform "wallet biopsies" on uninsured patients. Through these "wallet biopsies," the AHA's co-defendants' priorities are not necessarily on the appropriate healthcare treatment for the uninsured patient but rather on gouging the uninsured patient with exorbitantly inflated prices, in some cases up to 300 percent more than for insured patients.

Scruggs Law Firm
July 21, 2004

Press Release: Statement from the American Hospital Association on class action lawsuit—America's hospitals are about people taking care of people, often at the most vulnerable times in their life. That is the responsibility hospitals take seriously. Day in and day out. . . . This assault on community hospitals is misdirected and baseless—diverting the focus away from the real issue of how we as a nation are going to extend health care coverage to all Americans.

Dick Davidson
President of the American Hospital Association
July 21, 2004

How hospital performance data are presented is utterly and purposefully confusing. After first proposing a five-star rating system, the JACHO (Joint Commission on Accreditation of Healthcare Organizations) has turned to a grid of overall and separate scores. After tweaking, some stars have returned, though what they stand for now is anyone's guess. What payers, let alone hapless consumers, are supposed to do with this jumble is unknown but probably irrelevant.

Todd Sloane
Assistant managing editor/op-ed of *Modern Healthcare*
August 2, 2004

Everyone knows what a hospital is. It is where people go in a medical emergency; to have technologically sophisticated tests done to determine if their symptoms are indicative of a serious health problem; to have surgery or other procedures done; and so on. People generally do not think about hospitals unless they need to go to one because of a pressing health problem. When they do go, they are naturally preoccupied with the health problem that is causing them to be there. For purposes of this discussion we will be taking a broader view of hospitals. We will look at hospitals as organizational structures, and we will identify who owns them and who decides how they operate.

The first consideration is that hospitals are not all alike. Some are small community hospitals; some are very large and linked to other large organizations, such as medical schools. There are also highly specialized hospitals — for example, those that treat patients who only need physical rehabilitation. If you cannot quite see a master plan here, you are making the right interpretation. Hospitals have evolved to meet the needs of particular communities. The community they intend to serve is something they themselves decide. To understand how hospitals have evolved, let us begin with the first decade of the twentieth century.

First, it would be good to consider a number of other basic characteristics that distinguish hospitals one from another. The most basic difference stems from how long patients stay in the hospital. There are short-term-stay, "acute care" hospitals, and there are long-term hospitals. The majority of hospitals in this country are short-stay hospitals. Long-term hospitals mostly care for mental patients and rehabilitation patients. There are also long-term care facilities that are not hospitals but nursing homes. We will discuss them later in this chapter. Unless otherwise indicated, the discussion to follow refers to short-term, acute care hospitals.

It might be helpful to look first at some growth trends among hospitals. Counting the number of hospitals tells you something but leaves a lot unsaid about growth. A more precise indicator would also tell us whether individual hospitals are getting larger. There are various ways to measure the size of an organization, including a hospital: the number of employees, the gross annual budget, the number of branches it has established, the size of the geographic region it serves, and so on. The commonly agreed-on measure in this case is the number of beds. A hospital in a rural area might have fifty to seventy-five beds while a medical center hospital might have five hundred or more beds. As you might imagine, the size of a hospital determines the range of services it can offer, the size and expertise of its staff, the sophistication of the equipment it has available, its budget, and its organizational concerns.

Another basic distinguishing criterion is hospital ownership. It turns out that who owns a particular hospital makes a significant difference and is an issue that has inspired heated debate over the past few of decades. When the government reports hospital statistics, it begins by differentiating between federal government hospitals and nonfederal hospitals. Federally owned and funded hospitals are basically operated by the Veterans Administration for the exclusive use of veterans of the armed forces. All other hospitals fall into the nonfederal category, subdivided into three ownership categories: nonprofit, for profit (previously called proprietary), and state/local government.

Hospitals in the state and local government category are the easiest to recognize. They are usually named to clearly indicate that they are government sponsored—for example, Boston City Hospital, Los Angeles County Hospital, or University of Illinois Hospital. You realize, of course, that the state and local government hospitals are, in the broadest sense, not-for-profit organizations. They are typically referred to as public hospitals—that is, funded by the public through taxes—to distinguish them from hospitals that are privately funded. The same labeling is used to identify the sponsorship of other organizations in the health sector and out. Any organization that is supported by taxes is considered a public organization.

The nonprofit category is not always so easy to distinguish from the for-profit category. Small community hospitals and major teaching hospitals qualify as nonprofit hospitals. University-sponsored teaching hospitals usually, but not always, carry the name of the medical school that owns and operates them. Many other hospitals are loosely affiliated with medical schools, which themselves may be publicly or privately supported nonprofit organizations. Affiliation to a medical school allows a hospital to offer graduate medical education in the form of residency programs, in which persons who have already earned a medical doctor's degree (i.e., medical residents) carry out their postgraduate, practical, on-the-job medical training. Medical schools have more graduates than they can accommodate at the university hospital for residency training, which takes anywhere from three to five years, more if the doctor wishes to subspecialize. For this reason, university/teaching hospitals must develop ties to state, local, and "community" hospitals to provide places for medical students and residents to receive hands-on training.

The term *community hospital* has traditionally served as a catchall label for hospitals that are owned and operated for the benefit of the community as opposed to that of owners and investors. Such hospitals may have been established by religious orders, residents of a particular geographic community, or leading citizens within a particular community aiming to create a hospital to provide for their own religious or ethnic groups. The government has recently begun to use the *community* label more broadly to refer to all acute care hospitals regardless of ownership (as denoted in table 4.1).

The for-profit category includes hospitals that are privately owned and operated as profit-making enterprises. Historically, this label referred to hospitals that were owned by individuals, usually one or more doctors. As owners, they pocketed what they earned from running the hospital; they made all the decisions regarding general improvements, technological and cosmetic improvements, staff, and so on. They also paid taxes on any profits. This is a major distinction. Nonprofit hospitals are not taxed by the government. Proprietary hospitals of this kind have all but disappeared, although any that still exist would fall into this category. The label is now understood to mean hospitals that are owned by corporations (to make things more confusing, this is sometimes referred to as being "publicly owned" because many people are owners by virtue of investing in it). These hospitals aim to make a profit: they sell shares to stockholders, distribute profits to those who invest in the business, and pay taxes. Table 4.1 indicates growth trends in each of these categories since 1975.

Because counting the number of beds is generally considered to be a more accurate measure of hospital trends, table 4.2 reports the shift in the number of hospital beds between 1975 and 2001. As you can see, the total number of beds has been declining since 1975. However, it is the distribution of beds that policy makers were most interested in, especially the fact that the number of beds in for-profit hospitals continued to increase. We will get back to that observation shortly.

Table 4.1. Hospitals in the United States, 1975–2001

	1975	1995	2001
All hospitals	7,156	6,291	5,801
Federal	359	299	243
Community			
Nonprofit	3,322	3,09	2,998
For-profit	730	752	754
State/local	1,778	1,350	1,156

Source: "Hospitals, Beds, and Occupancy Rates, according to Type of Ownership and Size of Hospital: United States, Selected Years 1875–2001," *Health United States, 2003* (Washington, D.C.: U.S Department of Health and Human Services, Public Health Service, 2003), table 106.

Table 4.2. Distribution of Hospital Beds, 1975–2001

	1975		1995		2001	
All	1,465,828	100%	1,080,601	100%	987,440	100%
Federal	131,946	9	77,079	7	51,900	5
Nonfederal	1,333,882	91	1,003,522	93	935,540	95
Community	941,844	100%	872,736	100%	825,966	100%
Nonprofit	658,195	70	609,729	70	585,070	71
For-profit	73,495	8	105,737	12	108,718	13
State/local	210,154	22	157,270	18	132,178	16

Source: "Hospitals, Beds, and Occupancy Rates, according to Type of Ownership and Size of Hospital: United States, Selected Years 1875–2001," *Health United States, 2003* (Washington, D.C.: U.S Department of Health and Human Services, Public Health Service, 2003), table 106.

A BRIEF HISTORY OF HOSPITALS IN THE TWENTIETH CENTURY

Before the twentieth century, people avoided a hospital stay if they had any choice about it. Hospitals were essentially charitable organizations that provided basic care and housing for indigents who had no place else to go. Exactly how many hospitals there were in this country around the turn of the century is difficult to determine. According to one of the few estimates available, as of the mid-1880s, there were only 178.[1] People did not go into a hospital willingly because everyone knew that hospitals were dangerous places. One's chances of dying once you were in the hospital were excellent. Middle-class people certainly would not have paid to go there. Those who could afford it were treated in their own homes or the doctor's office. Many people also sought advice and remedies from the apothecary (pharmacist) and any number of other kinds of health practitioners.

While most people were reluctant to go into the hospital during the first two decades of the twentieth century, surgeons were beginning to find it more difficult to perform surgery outside of the hospital. They had begun to perform more kinds of surgery than they had been able to do even a few decades before, largely due to a range of technological advances. Anesthesia, which was initially developed in the 1840s, had become more effective and reliable. (Imagine what surgery was like before anesthesia! People died from the shock of being cut open even before they had a chance to develop an infection; if they survived, infection was, of course, very likely.) The value of antisepsis (a sterile surgical environment) was discovered in the 1860s and was now fully implemented. X-ray technology came into existence in the 1890s. As surgeons became more dependent on hospitals to perform surgical procedures, they also became more interested in setting standards that would improve the quality of hospital care.

Accordingly, in 1918 the American College of Surgeons began inspecting hospitals in an effort to ensure the public that hospitals were well equipped and that the doctors doing surgery were well qualified. They did so by encouraging doctors to assume greater responsibility for overseeing the work of their colleagues. They were especially concerned about preventing less-qualified or unethical colleagues from performing unnecessary surgery.[2] The medical profession as a whole, led by the most accomplished surgeons, improved the quality of care provided in hospitals by having pathologists perform autopsies on the patients who died in the hospital to determine whether the diagnosis was accurate and whether the surgery was truly necessary and, of course, done well. The public nature of the autopsy meant that surgeons had to be more careful about the surgeries they were performing because all doctors affiliated with the hospital were encouraged to attend autopsies as an excellent method to discuss cases and advance medical knowledge. Having colleagues discover that the surgeon was misdiagnosing patients and performing unnecessary surgery would certainly not be good for the surgeon's reputation.

To ensure that autopsies were in fact being carried out and that the privileges of doctors doing inappropriate surgeries were restricted, the American College of Surgeons encouraged doctors to become active members of the Medical Staff organization in the hospital. In short, doctors were encouraged to establish firm control over the day-to-day work taking place in hospitals.

Administrators of hospitals were well aware of the fact that their interests were not identical to those of surgeons or, for that matter, other physicians and other hospital personnel. They began organizing themselves into an association of their own. In 1899 they established the Association of Hospital Superintendents of the United States and Canada, which became the American Hospital Association (AHA) within the next few years. Over the next decade or so the AHA came around to the view that the surgeons were probably right, that raising hospital standards was important and that inspections were essential. However, the AHA did not have the resources or the power over hospitals to impose such inspections. The American College of Surgeons did have that power.

When hospitals were primarily charitable institutions, doctors contributed their services. They did so because hospitals provided them with interesting "clinical material"—that is, interesting cases. In other words, the patients were more likely to be in an advanced stage of disease because they did not have the money to obtain treatment earlier, often because the disease prevented them from working and thus impoverished them. There were a lot of very sick people who could not afford to see a doctor privately. So doctors volunteered their services in exchange for the opportunity to treat the interesting cases. As hospital care improved, middle-class patients began asking to be admitted to the hospital, indicating willingness to pay the doctor as well as the hospital for the care they would receive. Here we begin to see a pattern that would lead to hospitals beginning to depend on patients' paying for the hospitals' operating funds. Surgeons were in a position to funnel their paying patients to the hospital of their choice. Hospitals were left with little alternative but to accede to the surgeons' wishes—focusing on making the improvements that surgeons demanded, such as bigger and better surgical suites, more advanced equipment, and more staff.

The AHA first approached the American College of Surgeons around 1950 to explore the possibility of setting up a cooperative inspection program. Four organizations joined together to develop hospital accreditation standards: the AHA, the American College of Surgeons, the American Medical Association, and the American College of Physicians. By 1952 they had worked out standards and established a new organization, the Joint Commission on Hospital Accreditation, to carry out the inspections. The inspections were to be voluntary; hospitals would have to request them and would be charged for the costs of carrying them out. As of 1987, it became the Joint Commission on Accreditation of Healthcare Organizations (JCAHO), generally now referred to as the Joint Commission. The role of JCAHO is very obvious to everyone employed in a hospital, especially when the Joint Commission comes in to do an accreditation visit.

Hospitals continued to grow and expand during the first few decades of the twentieth century, until the end of the 1930s.[3] According to one of the first American Medical Association counts, there were approximately forty-three hundred hospitals in the country in 1928. Then the trend suddenly reversed. By 1935, the number dropped to four thousand. The drop is attributed to the Great Depression. Patients could not afford to go to a hospital; those who were taken there because it was an emergency could not pay for it; and many smaller hospitals did not survive. The hospitals that did survive could absorb such losses only because they were receiving support from especially dedicated and, in many cases, wealthy contributors. Some hospitals survived because of the support they received from religious orders or an entire ethnic community. The only other hospitals that survived the Depression were those operated by local governments.

The next major event that occurred in the twentieth century was World War II, and little changed in the hospital sector between the Depression and the end of the war. Once the war ended, however, the country experienced a period of adjustment that brought with it not only peace but a period of unprecedented prosperity. Because Americans did not, really could not, spend much on consumer goods during the war years, they suddenly found themselves much better off financially than they had been prior to the war. People wasted no time making up for what they had forgone during the war years. They got married, had babies, built new homes out in the suburbs, bought things for their homes, and purchased cars. With all this expansion, there was a need for new schools, new roads, and of particular relevance to this discussion, new hospitals. The Hill-Burton Act was passed in 1946 to support the construction and expansion of hospitals. The federal government matched the funds raised by the community for the purpose of building a new hospital or adding on to an existing one. The result was that established hospitals expanded and new community hospitals sprang up in rural areas and suburbs all across the country.

At this point we should consider whether there really was a need for so much more hospital construction or whether there could have been some other reason behind the urge to build and expand. Admittedly, the definition of "need" in this case has its own body of literature. For purposes of this discussion, there is something besides objective need involved. Many hospitals came into existence for symbolic reasons. They stood as a major source of pride to the community whether it was an ethnic, religious, or geographical community. The Hill-Burton Act provided the perfect opportunity to act on that sense of pride. It is also true that some urban hospitals were built by people who had good reason to believe that they were not welcome in hospitals operated by other groups, such as Jewish hospitals. Jewish doctors experienced discrimination when seeking privileges in hospitals run by others. Jewish patients felt better being treated by doctors who they felt would understand their cultural values. Similarly, Catholic hospitals offered the assurance that patients could practice their religion and that priests would be readily available to offer solace, hear confession, and offer last rites. Immigrants were concerned about being able to communicate and wanted to be able to speak their own languages in the hospitals. Finally, the newly established suburban communities were interested in proving that they could offer everything that the city could offer, only newer and better. (See the social construction of reality at work here? The people building hospitals were certain there was a need for all those new hospitals and new additions—perhaps not the kind of need that policy analysts were looking for, but as you can see, "need" is in the eyes of the beholder.) It goes without saying that poor people in poor neighborhoods could not and did not take advantage of the Hill-Burton funds. For this reason, new hospitals were not built in the many communities that really needed them.

Aside from community pride in the hospital, there is one other factor that coincidentally came into play just after World War II ended that fostered the expansion of hospitals. Synthesized penicillin came into existence during the late 1940s and became widely available by 1950. (Scientists knew about the value of penicillin in its original state—that is, mold and cobwebs. It took a while to identify the chemical formula so that it could be produced in volume and under antiseptic conditions.) The availability of penicillin would have a major effect on hospital expansion because this was the first time that hospitals could control infection with certainty. Before that time, drugs to control infection did exist, but none was as powerful as the new series of antibiotics, starting with penicillin.

THE HISTORY OF HOSPITALS OVER THE LAST FIVE DECADES

Starting in the second half of the twentieth century, it seems that people were not only more willing to go into the hospital but were prepared to stay there for days. However, even at that time, staying in the hospital was not a minor expense. So who paid for people to luxuriate in the hospital for days? The answer is health insurance, initially Blue Cross, later commercial insurance, and as of 1965 Medicare and Medicaid (in short, the former is for the elderly, and the latter is for the poor; see chapter 7 for a more comprehensive discussion of health insurance).

The enactment of Medicare and Medicaid turns out to be a really big event for the future of U.S. hospitals and health care in general. The two programs guaranteed payment on behalf of those who had been least likely to be hospitalized because they could not afford it. That brought in a lot of "new business" to hospitals causing hospitals to grow and expand to accommodate increasing demand for health care services. (If talk about the business of health care delivery makes you think that things are finally going to be orderly and efficient, you are going to like what happens over the next few decades; if talk about the health care business makes you uncomfortable, prepare yourself: this is just the beginning. Hospitals and health care organizations are about to become *big business*.) The expenditures on hospital care went from $9 billion in 1960 to over $451 billion in 2001.[4]

From the perspective of hospitals, Medicare (and to a lesser extent Medicaid) would be providing a steady—and, more important, reliable—stream of funding from this time forward. By 1965, the government was already providing around 38 percent of the funding for hospital care (which includes various subsidies, research funds, and so on); by 2002, the government was providing just under 60 percent of the funding.[5] You know the old saying "He who pays the piper calls the tune"? The federal government has very little competition when it decides that it wants to call a particular tune. Here are two of the tunes it called from the beginning using the Medicare program as its vehicle for exclusive request of a song.

The government wanted some assurance that government funds would be going to good, as opposed to fly-by-night, hospitals. Therefore, the government decreed that Medicare funds could only go to hospitals that were accredited by the JCAHO (remember, this is the voluntary association created to upgrade standards). That not only gave the Joint Commission increased power, but it eliminated hospitals that could not successfully pass a review by the Joint Commission because they could not compete with hospitals that could advertise this stamp of approval.

The second tune was dedicated to Blue Cross–Blue Shield. The government was not about to set up its own bureaucracy to administer the Medicare program. Instead, it agreed to pay an administrative fee to organizations that were already processing health insurance claims. It seemed like a good idea to give that responsibility to an insurance company that was a nonprofit organization rather than one that would make a profit on public funds spent by the government. In time, the for-profit insurance companies convinced the government that they could provide the same services for less. That was an argument that appealed to the government and was popular with the public. Insurance carriers, who bid on providing this service for the lowest fee, now administer Medicare, generally on a state-by-state basis.

After the first two or three years, the government realized that Medicare costs would not drop, as policy analysts had expected. Policy analysts who projected costs had reasoned that a backlog of untreated illness would push up the initial costs of Medicare and Medicaid but that once that backlog was addressed, costs would drop. However, costs showed no sign of falling. The government did not take major steps to reduce costs until 1983, which is when diagnostic-related groups (DRGs) were introduced. The government developed a reimbursement schedule based on the diagnoses with which patients were admitted to the hospital. Hospitals were fully aware that this was coming and knew that the government was using the data that the hospitals themselves were submitting in order to receive Medicare reimbursements to construct the schedule. Amazingly, all possible diagnostic categories were subsumed into 467 categories, plus a few more catchall categories. The system was set up so that the government would pay X amount of money per diagnostic category (1 of the 476) per Medicare patient admission. Private insurance companies did not change their reimbursement arrangements in response to the introduction of DRGs, at least not immediately. However, over the decade of the 1990s, private insurance companies adopted the DRG reimbursement schedule, and Medicaid programs in most states did too.

If the hospital could do whatever was necessary for less than the DRG payment for particular procedures or services, it got to keep the extra funds. If the funds were insufficient, the hospital simply had to find a way to deal with that. Hospitals did find ways to deal with it. One was to increase charges to patients covered by private insurance. Another way was to begin cutting back on the number of days (length of stay) a person stayed in the hospital.

A number of factors were coming into play at the same time that had an impact on the length of stay in the hospital. Surgical techniques had been improving all along; more laser surgery was being used (which is less invasive and may be done on an outpatient basis); and everyone agreed that it was better for the patient to go home to more familiar and comforting surroundings (where there was less chance of contracting new strains of infection that are hospital based). The reason for paying attention to length of stay is the impact this has on hospital occupancy rates. If people stayed in the hospital for fewer days, that would leave beds empty. If this trend continued, hospitals would have to take beds out of service permanently, and that is exactly what happened. Some hospitals had such a low "census," or occupancy rate, that they could no longer survive, which explains the decline in hospitals and hospital beds over the last two decades.

The introduction of DRGs marked an important turning point in the operations of hospitals regardless of ownership. Consider the fact that, before DRGs, Medicare paid hospitals on the basis of charges, not costs. In other words, whatever the hospital charged was what Medicare paid. The government created DRGs because many critics repeatedly pointed out that paying on a charge basis, rather than a cost basis, was one of the main reasons behind the escalation of costs. They argued that hospitals could and should become more efficient and accountable for how they were spending public funds. Hospitals had no alternative but to become more efficient.

Hospitals came up with yet another way to make up for the loss they sustained because of tighter Medicare controls in response to DRGs. They were already reducing the length of stay; all they had to do was extend that idea. They simply admitted patients for less than a full day (i.e., less than twenty-four hours). Since DRGs cover inpatient care but not outpatient care, hospitals could charge rates that were not so closely monitored. This practice explains why hospitals began building freestanding, outpatient clinics both near and far from the parent hospital.

The declining length of stay plus the increase in outpatient facilities contributed to the decline in the number of hospital beds during the 1980s. This trend, in turn, explains another closely related phenomenon. By the late 1980s, the patients being admitted to the hospital were too seriously ill to be treated on an outpatient basis. In other words, hospitals were now admitting sicker patients requiring more personal attention and more technologically sophisticated care. This manifested itself in two diametrically opposed trends that actually make perfect sense when you think about it. First, the ratio of staff to patients was steadily increasing; second, personnel costs were steadily declining compared to other hospital costs, which were skyrocketing. What accounts for rising hospital costs is not so difficult to understand once you start thinking about all the new technology that hospitals have invested in. This includes diagnostic and monitoring equipment, such as CT (computerized axial tomography) scanners, MRI (magnetic resonance imaging) equipment, and the computers that compile and analyze all the information that the diagnostic equipment produces. All those machines are enormously expensive, and they are replaced every other year or so as newer, improved versions are released. Every patient most certainly wants the most recent version of any diagnostic instrument available, and your doctor certainly feels that way, too; that, among other things (such as the threat of malpractice suits for using outdated equipment) convinces the hospital that staying current is a wise investment.

Clearly, hospitals could make stringent efforts to become more cost conscious when buying new equipment. However, since one of the main ways hospitals promote themselves is on the basis of having the latest technology, it is difficult to see why they would be interested in cutting back on all that highly sophisticated technological equipment and the highly paid staff required to operate it. To cover these costs, hospitals increasingly began relying on a traditional funding mechanism—namely, the "sliding scale," meaning the rich paid more than the nonrich. In its more recent incarnation, it became known as "cost-shifting"—that is, charging privately insured patients more than those whose bills were paid by public insurance. More recently, hospitals have been entering into contractual arrangements with some private insurance companies but not others. Anyone who is not included in such arrangements is charged more. Whether they are actually able to pay what they are charged is another matter.

Unfair? Hospital representatives say that they must take care of persons who carry no insurance but run up high costs. Where are they supposed to get the funds to cover that? Laws passed in 1986 prevent hospitals from turning away patients who are uninsured and unable to pay for care.[6] Hospitals are allowed to stabilize such patients and send them off to the nearest government-supported hospital. However, sometimes this involves emergency surgery and days spent in the most expensive part of the hospital, the "intensive care" unit. Surgical patients who are admitted to the hospital for a planned, routine surgery typically only spend a short time there. Patients who are involved in serious accidents or have multiple gun-shot wounds stay much longer. There is no public funding to cover the costs of caring for patients who require this kind of intensive care but are poor and have no insurance to cover it. Over the last couple of decades, additional funds called "disproportionate share hospital payments" have been legislated to help cover the costs incurred by hospitals that care for large numbers of poor and uninsured patients. However, administrators of such hospitals say that they continue to struggle to make ends meet.

HOSPITALS AT THE TURN OF THE TWENTY-FIRST CENTURY

Policy makers who focus on the hospital sector of the health care system have been following a number of developments for the last quarter century. The steady expansion of for-profit hospitals came under increased scrutiny during this period. For-profit hospital corporations had been growing at an unexpectedly fast rate. The representatives of these corporations argued that what they were doing was socially beneficial because it put pressure on nonprofit hospitals to be more efficient, which they said would bring down prices. Critics countered by arguing that the aggressive form of competition introduced by the for-profit hospital corporations went too far, that it made it more difficult for the poor and uninsured to receive care because the nonprofit hospitals could not afford to provide "charity" care and keep their doors open. They said that competition brought downsizing to hospitals, which translated into laying off the most experienced and therefore most expensive nurses and hiring less expensive, easily replaced "technicians" trained to do very specific tasks (e.g., take blood pressure or give shots). The problem, the critics said, is that bringing in less-skilled personnel was increasing the risk of mistakes—medication errors, inability to recognize disease indicators, carelessness about disposal of infectious materials, and so on.

A good indicator of public concern was the pressure it put on legislators to pass laws to prevent patients from being discharged prematurely (i.e., earlier than what the public thought appropriate) or, as policy analysts put it, to prevent their falling victim to the "quicker and sicker" cycle. By the end of 1996, twenty-nine states had passed laws governing "early discharge" to prevent women who had just had a baby from being discharged in less than two days or those who had a mastectomy from being discharged the same day.[7] The laws were actually directed at the insurance companies responsible for restrictions on length of stay. We will get back to this topic in later chapters. For now, let's just say that health policy types see this as a very strange way to deal with the problem of quality of care. Do we expect legislators to pass laws to cover every possible concern about hospital care expressed by the public?

The major problem, according to some observers, has been that the commitment to business practices led to mergers and buyouts of entire hospital corporations. Hospitals began acting more as other businesses, interested in increasing their profits by focusing on cutting expenditures—the old "leaner and meaner" story. As tables that appeared earlier in this chapter show, the number of for-profit hospitals increased steadily. To survive in this environment, nonprofit hospitals began to adopt aggressive business practices similar to those used by for-profit hospitals. By the end of the twentieth century, it became more difficult to identify the differences between for-profit hospitals and nonprofit hospitals.

Whether the changes that took place in the hospital sector have been good for patients, health sector personnel, and society as a whole has been the subject of controversy for quite some time. We will return in later chapters to the question of whether increased reliance on a business model for running hospitals has been beneficial or detrimental, for now the basic elements of the argument are these. Those in favor of the continued growth of the for-profit hospital sector say it is about time that hospitals learned to apply basic business practices. They say that the growth of the for-profits has introduced better management techniques, reduced costs, improved service, and so forth. Those who are opposed say the for-profits skim off the richest, healthiest patients; do almost no research, no medical education; and have as their primary goal financial gain that benefits hospital executives and shareholders. The critics argue that the health care delivery system should not be making a profit on the members of society who have the misfortune of being sick.

Which side is right? Depends on your perspective. The answer boils down to whether you think recent trends are more beneficial to society as a whole or to that portion of society that is getting rich from investments in the health sector.

OTHER HEALTH CARE ORGANIZATIONS

Applying one of the basic differentiating characteristics used in discussing hospitals, we can differentiate some other health care organizations by whether they care for patients who are ambulatory (to ambulate is to walk) or bedridden. Ambulatory patients may receive care at clinics, now more often called health centers, which can be freestanding or attached to a hospital. Patients can be acutely but temporarily ill or chronically ill; in both cases, they receive health care services on an outpatient basis for whatever time it takes, whether long term or short term. Long-term-care patients, who are no longer able to get to the hospital or clinic on a regular basis without a great deal of assistance, may end up being admitted to a facility to receive care as inpatients. Long-term-care facilities are generally privately owned, often operated as for-profit organizations. While most rely on Medicare and Medicaid funds, the facilities themselves are typically not government owned.

Long-term care, both inpatient and outpatient, has been attracting a considerable amount of attention over the last few decades.[8] The reason is perfectly clear—fear that this will turn into a serious problem. You know that the baby boom generation is moving right along toward their golden years. As the boomers develop health problems associated with aging, they are expected to break the bank. The list of threatened institutions is lengthy: social security, Medicare, nursing home care, and all associated services required by the elderly. The expected increase in the number of aged who require nursing home care plus the increasing number of severely disabled younger people requires serious attention and planning.

Added to the increasing number of people who will need nursing home care because of the problems associated with aging is the devastation caused by chronic illness in younger populations—for example, paralysis due to spinal injury, mental problems, and HIV/AIDS. Finally, the fact that modern medicine can perform miracles in saving people who would not have survived years ago does not necessarily mean that those who are saved can lead normal, healthy lives. Many require extensive care for years.

The over-sixty-five population is, however, of greatest concern to policy makers because of the numbers involved. Only about 4 percent to 5 percent of this population is in a nursing home at any point. The explanation is that they usually do not stay in nursing homes for very long. The average length of stay is approximately 80 days, but for persons over eighty-five it goes up to 145 days. The problem is that even a short stay is expensive, $4,000 to $5,000 per month. Nursing homes are classified as skilled nursing facilities (SNFs), which provide the full range of health services that a convalescent patient might need; and intermediate nursing facilities (INFs), which provide less-extensive health-related services, including rehabilitation, personal care, and social services. Medicare, more often Medicaid, reimburses for care provided by the facilities. A growing number of people need custodial care not because they are ill but because they are frail, forgetful, and not fully able to manage on their own. This kind of care is not funded.

Home health care has been supported, in fact promoted, albeit with some trepidation, by the government as a good alternative to nursing home care. The reason that home health care is not likely to be promoted even more enthusiastically is that it poses a potential cost problem that is interesting to reflect upon. Home health care is much less expensive than nursing home care because people stay in their own homes and health workers go in for a few hours at a time. Also, virtually everyone prefers to stay in his or her own home. The problem is the fear that too many people will opt for this form of care. Traditionally, wives, daughters, and other female relatives provided such care out of sense of duty. Now that the majority of women are not staying home, the government is concerned that it will have to pick up the bill. For now, the costs do not seem to be rising too rapidly, but this cost item is being carefully monitored.

Hospices are another interesting innovation. For years, critics said terminally ill patients did not have to be in the hospital. It was too expensive; it put the patient through unnecessary pain and aggravation; it was a bad idea all around. Hospices promised to provide the patient with comfort and relief from pain, rather than aggressive intervention. The result was expected to be less expensive. As it turns out, the kind of care patients are receiving is pretty much what was anticipated. Most people think it is excellent. The problem is that it has not reduced costs very much.

CONCLUSION

As is obvious, we have encountered many kinds of issues in this chapter. One's conclusions depend on the questions that one wishes to address. Working backward, we can ask, Are alternatives to hospitalization worth developing? The general consensus seems to be yes, they are. However, how we can accomplish that objective is not at all clear, which is where institution building comes in. Since there is no blueprint, anyone who has a plan is trying to institute it. Will that work? No one knows with certainty, but since we do not know how else to do it, we will most likely continue along the same path.

How about the future of hospitals? The questions here largely revolve around who we want to see operating them. Asking who is best suited or who will do the best job for us is, at bottom, a matter of perspective on the benefits of competition and private sector ownership versus dependence on nonprofit organizations plus greater government involvement and oversight. This is not something that people debate without emotion. Those who are most closely involved tend to be believers in one approach or the other. Rarely do you find people sitting on the fence. Even if you have not come to this debate with strong feelings about this question already, by the time you finish this book, you too will likely be taking sides.

Theoretical perspectives are useful in explaining "where people are coming from" when they enter such debates. Theoretical perspectives do not, however, provide clear answers to the questions raised in such discussions, nor are they designed to do so. To begin with, the functionalist and conflict theory perspectives do not match the two sides of the debate, if only because one side is not as well articulated as the other. At the heart of the controversy is the question of whether health care organizations are like other organizations that produce and sell goods and services or whether they are somehow different.

Where the conflict theorists stand on this point is perfectly clear. They say that health care delivery organizations are special, that they should not be operated for profit. They argue that the misfortune of others should not provide an opportunity to further enrich the rich and powerful in society. And they say that health care is too important to treat as just another commodity that can be traded on the market, like pork bellies, or as a product that is purchased as a matter of preference, like a breakfast cereal.

Functionalists are neither seen nor heard discussing these points. This is not to say that the other side of the argument about the nature of health care organizations is not being vigorously represented. It is just that the people who are taking the lead are economists, who do not employ the same labels as sociologists to identify themselves as functionalists or conflict theorists. We will discuss what they have to say when we discuss health care reform in chapter 11. There are, however, many more topics to cover before we do that. Health care occupations is the topic we address next.

NOTES

1. E. H. L. Corwin, *The American Hospital* (New York: Commonwealth Fund, 1946).

2. Rosemary Stevens, *In Sickness and in Wealth* (New York: Basic Books, 1989).

3. "Hospital Service in the United States," *Journal of the American Medical Association* 106 (April 3, 1925): 1009; "Hospital Service in the United States," *Journal of the American Medical Association* 106 (March 7, 1935): 792.

4. "National Health Expenditures, Average Annual Percent Change, and Percent Distribution according to Type of Expenditure: United States, Selected Years 1960–2001," *Health United States, 2003* (Washington D.C.: U.S. Department of Health and Human Services, Public Health Service, 2003), table 115.

5. "National Health Care Expenditures, Hospital Care Expenditures Aggregated and Per Capita Amounts, Percent Distribution and Average Annual Percent Change by Source of Funds: Selected Calendar Years 1990–2013" (Baltimore, Md.: Centers for Medicare & Medicaid Services, 2003), table 6.

6. The Combined Budget Reconciliation Act of 1985 (COBRA)—which prohibits hospitals receiving Medicare funds from transferring unstable patients and women in active labor until they are stabilized—went into effect on August 1, 1986.

7. Eugene Declercq and Diana Simmes, "The Politics of 'Drive-Through Deliveries': Putting Early Postpartum Discharge on the Legislative Agenda," *Milbank Quarterly* 75 (1997): 175–202.

8. Alice Rivlin and Joshua Wiener, *Caring for the Disabled Elderly* (Washington D.C.: Brookings Institution, 1988).

5

The Division of Labor in the Health Care Delivery System

America's physicians have never looked to government as their savior. However, while they were guarding their flanks against "big government" and its power, they were blind-sided by employers who discovered they could bargain with insurers over benefits and premiums, by insurers who—responding to employers—exercised control over issues of productivity, requiring more "output" at lower reimbursement, and by managed care organizations who organized delivery systems that tried to preempt the physician's independence and exercise of clinical judgement. Although American medicine may fear government's exercise of arbitrary power, government is accountable. The real danger lies in the faceless, inexorable, profit-motivated market, an institution from which there is no appeal.

Rashi Fein
Journal of the American Medical Association
August 13, 2003

Nurse understaffing is ranked by the public and physicians as one of the greatest threats to patient safety in U.S. hospitals.

Linda Aiken, Sean Clarke,
Robyn Cheung, Douglas Sloane, and Jeffrey Silber
Journal of the American Medical Association
September 24, 2003

"The hardest thing is staying ahead of the curve of absurdity. We'll joke about one thing then we'll see it in the *Wall Street Journal* a week later. . . ." Dr. Levy and Dr. LaGana don't pretend to have the answers to health care's woes. They want "Damaged Care" to encourage physicians and others to take leadership roles to improve health care. They hope to leave you

laughing. And thinking. . . . Back on stage, the two doctors are singing
"That's Cost Containment" to the tune of "That's Entertainment."
Tell patients that they've overstayed
Tell the docs they cannot be paid
Fire three nurses, hire an aide
That's cost containment

Damon Adams
American Medical News
August 2, 2004

Consider the categories of people who have some connection to the health
care delivery system. Just to name a few participants, there are doctors, patients, nurses, therapists, technicians, and administrators. There are providers
and consumers. There are specialists, family practitioners, medical social
workers, chiropractors, counselors, plus all those people whose titles are not
easily recognizable but whose responsibility it is to arrange for treatments to
be scheduled, approved, and paid for. Then there are all those people who offer health care services but who are not part of what is generally recognized to
be the mainstream health care delivery system. In most but not all cases, they
stand outside of the mainstream by choice. We will focus on them in the next
chapter. In this chapter, we will discuss the occupational groups that are generally recognized as integral to the mainstream health care delivery system.

It is not always exactly clear what some health care staffers do. The people
who work in hospitals generally know right away. They do not have to recognize the person. They can tell just by looking at what the person is wearing. The most easily distinguishable is the loose-fitting green or blue two-
piece outfit that resembles pajamas. We all know from watching hospital
television shows that those things are called "scrubs," or scrub suits. They are
worn in the surgical suite by doctors and nurses. We also know that this outfit is symbolic of a high-status activity.

The status designated by other kinds of garments may be less familiar. Senior medical staff members wear coats with their names sewn on the pocket.
The coats have traditionally been white; now they are sometimes gray. Interns
and residents wear something of similar design except that it is only suit-
jacket length but does have their name on the pocket. Most other staff members see their names on plastic name tags, which they are expected to wear at
all times. Then there were the neat white shirtwaist dress and cap that distin-
guished nurses from everyone else, which now only appear in old movies.
Nurses are more likely to be seen wearing loose-fitting smocks. These too are
shorter than the long coat worn by doctors. A few decades ago, other members of nursing departments—ward clerks, for example—were expected to

wear a specific color of smock that indicated job responsibility as well as rank and educational preparation. Volunteers wear smocks. There was a time when young women volunteers, known as "candy stripers," wore easy-to-identify, prim, pink and white-stripped shirtwaist dresses. It seems that there is a correlation between the length and style of the garment and the status of the wearer. If this is not immediately apparent to you when you visit a hospital, the reason is that emphasizing status gradations so boldly is not nearly as socially acceptable now as it was a few decades ago. Status gradations in hospitals are just as important, maybe more so, but the outward symbols that proclaim status have become less obvious.

Job titles or labels are important, even when the length and color of the designated outfit one wears to work is not at issue. For example, would you prefer to define yourself as a "patient" or as a "consumer" of health care services? You might wonder what the difference is, but the two labels carry very different connotations, which bring with them a whole set of unstated meanings that establish the framework from which this discussion proceeds. We will return in a later chapter to the focus on "consumer-driven" health care that has recently been heavily promoted.

The introduction of such labels provides a good example of how the process of constructing reality affects people's understandings of the facts with which they are operating. The imagery associated with the *consumer* label connotes someone who is interested in shopping for the best deal, who knows what he or she is looking for, who expects to get what he or she pays for—namely, good value for the money. The word *patient* generally does not immediately bring to mind shopping behavior. For most people it brings to mind a person who has a health concern that he or she would like to have checked out. It suggests health care–seeking behavior aimed at getting the best treatment rather than the best buy. The two sets of images are not necessarily mutually exclusive. However, you must admit that there are some telling differences here. From a sociological perspective, those subtle differences are worth attending to because they frame, even define, society's perception of reality.

The number and kinds of people, as well as the tasks they perform, have expanded tremendously since the beginning of the last century. It is not much of an exaggeration to say that at the beginning of the twentieth century, there were only three positions in the hospital: doctor, nurse, and aide. The doctor's job was to diagnose and treat the patient. Nurses were responsible for keeping the patient clean and comfortable; aides, who may not have been called aides at the time, were responsible for making the room clean and comfortable. Doctors' offices had no support staff. Sometimes, the doctor's wife would help with the bills, and, of course, someone had to clean the office.

How things have changed! Well over 9 percent of Americans now work in the health care sector and do many more complex tasks than anyone could have imagined even thirty or forty years ago.[1] This raises a number of basic questions: Where did all those jobs come from? Who is in charge of creating new jobs? How does the work get divided? Scholars who study such issues would ask what the division of labor is and what the factors involved in creating that conformation are.

There are some 450 occupational titles involved; obviously, we can only discuss a small number of them. We will focus on doctors as opposed to all the other "allied health occupations" because doctors have the final authority when it comes to diagnosis and treatment and because doctors are licensed to prescribe medications and perform surgery. With very few exceptions that is the exclusive right of doctors. (An exception to this rule involves advanced practice nurses—e.g., nurse practitioners, nurse anesthetists, and nurse mid-wives. Practice privileges vary from state to state.) Traditionally, doctors have been able to charge a fee for their services. Most health care workers are salaried, meaning that they must answer to the employer, usually the hospital, not to the patient.

DOCTORS

There is no question that medicine is an occupation that is associated with high status and high income. Some Americans have come to believe that doctors' status and income are too high. It seems ironic that doctors were held in higher regard in the past, when they could do far less for their patients, than they are today, when they can deliver nearly miraculous cures and treatments. However, this is the judgment that many Americans are making. Perhaps we can get a clearer picture of the reasons behind the shift in social attitudes by examining the medical profession's development over time.

Let's begin by considering the fate of medicine as an occupation over the last century.[2] If we go back to the late nineteenth century, we see that there were a number of competing explanations for the existence of ill health, even death, all represented by groups of practitioners who offered particular kinds of treatments based on those explanations. There were many kinds of practitioners: hydropaths, who used water to soothe but, more often than not, to aggressively heat up or cool down the body; naturopaths, who are interested in preventing disease and use natural herbal remedies to treat symptoms; chiropractors, who treat most ailments using back manipulation and massage; homeopaths, who believe in treating "like symptoms with like" in an effort to attain stability and bring comfort; osteopaths, or D.O.'s (doctors of osteopathy), who subscribe to the idea that the backbone is the body's control center and that its strength is central to good health (they have come closest to the beliefs espoused by mainstream medicine over the last half-century and are now considered to be mainstream doctors); and, allopaths, who were engaging in aggressive interventions, such as bloodletting and giving emetics to induce vomiting, and if they were not successful, they simply applied more of the same treatment.

Interestingly, of all these groups it was the allopaths who became more closely allied with science. By the beginning of the twentieth century, allopathic medicine had firmly established itself as the mainstream form of medicine. The other practitioners did not exactly disappear, although some were absorbed by allopathic mainstream medicine while others came to be defined as unscientific and lost ground in competing for patients. Practitioners other than mainstream medical doctors now offer what has been called "alternative medicine" or, more recently, "complementary" and "integrative" medicine. We will focus on these practitioners in the next chapter.

So what is it about allopathic medicine that made it scientific? And why did that allow the allopaths to win the battle of competing explanations for illness and death (i.e., morbidity and mortality, respectively)? Being "scientific" within the context of late-nineteenth-century allopathic medicine simply means that the explanations and ultimately the treatments could be substantiated. The allopaths could predict the course of disease with and without treatment. The same outcome was true from one instance or one person to another. They verified their diagnoses by doing autopsies. (This not only identified surgeons who were misdiagnosing patients, as mentioned in the preceding chapter, but allowed other doctors to compare the symptoms outlined in the patient's file to the effect on the organs involved.) They built up a body of knowledge and learned to apply it. Basically, an increasing number of people began to believe in allopaths' explanations as evidence of their success began to accumulate. Or, if you prefer, the allopaths made every effort to make sure people heard about their successes and were impressed by them.

The larger context of this period is worth reflecting on. This revolution was happening at about the time that Americans suddenly became convinced that science was the way to go in all areas of life. During the first decade of the twentieth century there was talk about scientific solutions for unlikely pursuits such as housewifery (i.e., housekeeping) and for popular ones (in some circles) such as management. The growth of confidence in scientific medicine was not a unique phenomenon but rather a part of a broader shift in social values and expectations.

Accordingly, when the allopaths (hereafter referred to as doctors, or M.D.'s) focused on one area of practice and developed greater experience and expertise, they received high praise and recognition. Developing expertise was seen as a very good thing. Those who could afford it were eager to be treated by medical experts. True, the majority of people could not afford the kind of care medical experts could provide. They relied on home remedies and elixirs provided by the corner druggist. The doctors who were interested in becoming experts, or more precisely specialists, were engaging in behavior that was consistent with the society's values. Admittedly, these were the values espoused by the elite in the society, which the middle class emulated and which the poor pretty much ignored because they could not afford any kind of doctor, let alone care by a specialist.

MEDICAL SPECIALIZATION

Let's consider the matter of specialization in more detail. According to the prevailing popular wisdom, doctors are eager to specialize in order to make more money. Perhaps. But, like a lot of things in life, a closer examination reveals that the picture is more complicated than one blanket explanation can cover. Also, the matter of motivations attributed to whole categories of people is really stretching scientific analysis beyond the limit.

It is worth going back to the late nineteenth and early twentieth century to get the full picture. The first specialty to emerge was ophthalmology (medical and surgical treatment of the eye). One reason for this might be that new and better tools were becoming available during the latter half of the nineteenth century, making it easier to detect abnormalities in the eye. By the late nineteenth century, there were small groups of doctors meeting to discuss their observations about the eye and the new tools they were just getting accustomed to using. They were the ones who decided to establish a specialty of their own. Why do that, you ask? To make more money? Why not just put up a sign announcing that they were specialists and charge more anyway? Was money the only motivation here? A closer look at how people entered into most occupations might help answer that question.

At the turn of the century a doctor announced his or her occupation by putting up a sign declaring the kinds of work he or she was prepared to do. City directories, which were much like our current telephone books, listed people's occupations. You could list any occupation you wanted, qualified or not. People could, and did, simply pick up, move, and start doing different kinds of work whenever it suited them. This might be surprising, but there was strong opposition to all forms of licensure until the last decades of the nineteenth century. When the movement to institute licensure took hold in the 1880s, it occurred on a state-by-state basis. Today, states continue to control licensure, and a license from one state may not be honored in another state.

Returning to our ophthalmology example, why would an individual be interested in developing an official specialty designation? After all, anyone who had a medical degree, and in some cases those who did not, could put up a sign saying that he or she specialized in treating diseases of the eye. Obviously, no one would want to let just anybody treat his or her eyes, let alone cut into them. But wasn't insisting that practitioners be required to have a medical license enough? It is not hard to understand that people would want to be assured that they were going to practitioners who really had the best skills at the time. The doctors who were restricting their practices to treating people's eye problems and meeting with colleagues to upgrade their knowledge on a regular basis did in fact know more about eye disease than anyone else. They really did have greater expertise in their field, but there was no sure way for them to distinguish themselves from anyone else who laid claim to the label of *eye specialist.*

It was the experts in treatment of eye diseases who decided to institute specialty "certification." The doctors themselves set up training programs and a qualifying test for the purpose of recognizing new practitioners as qualified specialists. That is how ophthalmology became the first certified specialty in 1916. As an aside, how do you think other physicians reacted to this event? They were generally pleased, as most reputable doctors were not interested in treating eye problems because the eye is such a complex organ.

Other areas of specialization followed. The majority of doctors did not choose to specialize. They identified themselves as "physicians and surgeons" throughout the first half of the twentieth century. Why, then, are there so many specialists now? It must be the money, right? We can look for the answer in the sequence of events that emerged from the time when the first specialty came into existence, in 1916, to the last decade of the twentieth century.

World War II stands as a major turning point. The wartime draft made a major impression on doctors. It seems that specialists entered into military service as captains while the general practitioners entered as lieutenants. Obviously, with the higher rank of captain came higher pay and other privileges. Not the least of the privileges was the fact that captains were assigned to hospitals away from the battleground, while the lieutenants were assigned to field hospitals at the front. A parallel trend was taking off at home.

Because wartime wages were frozen, the only way that companies could make themselves more attractive to prospective employees, who were in short supply, was to offer better benefits. That provided insurance companies with an attractive new market. Insurance companies could not operate without standardizing the fees they would pay for the medical services. Before this time, doctors pretty much charged what they decided to charge depending on where they practiced and how much their patients were able to pay. It was the insurance companies, which set up standardized fee schedules, that set the pattern of paying specialists at a higher rate than general practitioners.

Toward the end of World War II, there is the effect of the GI Bill to consider. One of the big rewards for military service during the war was free education upon return. A large number of veterans took advantage of this benefit, including those who already had a medical degree. They went on to get more education and experience better suited to treating patients who were not war casualties. With more training, they became eligible for certification as specialists. Some went on to take specialty certification exams. Many others announced that they were specialists based on the fact that they completed all the requirements and were qualified to take certification tests, even if they did not actually take that final step. How did society react? Clearly, people were eager to be treated by doctors who had the most knowledge and expertise—that is, those who were trained as specialists.

A central feature of life in the United States from the mid-1960s through the early 1970s—in addition to the Vietnam War, antiwar protests, and the civil rights movement—was the increased role the government was playing in civilian life. The government was funneling considerable sums of money into social programs of all kinds (education, housing, and so forth), with medical research receiving a large share of those funds. Research monies went to medical schools for the purpose of carrying out specific kinds of research. There was an explosion of scientific knowledge. Medical students were not at all sure that they could learn everything they needed to know. Specialization allowed them to learn more about one subject area. Furthermore, medical students were heavily influenced by the excitement surrounding the work of specialists and superspecialists. Medical faculty served as impressive role models for new trainees.[3]

In the meantime, with all the emphasis on specialization, general practitioners were really becoming unhappy. They were being paid less than specialists for providing the same services. Patients were self-referring themselves to specialists because they perceived specialists to be more highly qualified. The general practitioners decided that they were tired of being treated as second-class citizens. They decided to make themselves specialists in "family practice," and that is exactly what happened in 1971. Family practice became a specialty just like any other medical or surgical specialty. This meant that after finishing medical school and receiving their M.D., doctors would continue their training in a specialized residency program. Before this time, a person with an M.D. was required to complete a one-year internship program to obtain a license to practice (which is granted by the states). From 1971 forward, all M.D.'s would be required to complete residencies lasting at least three years, more to become even more highly specialized. In short, as of 1971, there were no more general practitioners coming out of American medical schools. Currently, all doctors completing their education in the United States are specialists. We now refer to doctors who are primarily responsible for a patient's health as "primary care" practitioners, or as the latest acronym would have it, as PCPs. This includes internists, pediatricians, and family practitioners. The American Medical Association (AMA) also includes obstetricians and gynecologists, even though others qualified to count primary care physicians generally do not include them.

MEDICAL ERROR AND MALPRACTICE

Just about the time that the general practice option was abolished, Americans began to register increasing dissatisfaction with their health care arrangements. They complained that doctors were no longer interested in the whole person; they were only interested in treating parts of the person, and they were doing it only for the money (that old, familiar refrain). This explains, in part, the rapidly rising rate at which patients sue their doctors for malpractice. When the majority of doctors were general practitioners and worked in the community where their patients lived, the neighborhood residents got to know the doctor. When they needed to see the doctor, they went with the added comfort of an existing sense of familiarity and trust. That is not the case when patients see a doctor for a specific problem on a one-time basis. When things go wrong, it is a lot easier to sue that doctor, who is, after all, a stranger.

A number of factors may be contributing to what has come to be viewed as a malpractice crisis during the early years of the twenty-first century. Some observers believe that the widely quoted report on the rate of medical error has something to do with it. The matter of medical error came to public attention in 1999 when the Institute of Medicine (IOM; the quasi-government organization created to advise the nation on health issues) reported that forty-four thousand to ninety-eight thousand people die in hospitals due to preventable error per year.[4] While the numbers were actively disputed, everyone agreed that error reduction was a highly laudable objective. It is also true that the IOM report clearly stated that the rate of error was due to systemic failure rather than malpractice on the part of doctors. Nevertheless, it is possible that the report prompted some dissatisfied patients to sue.

It is hard to know the extent to which the number of malpractice suits has been rising because fewer bad doctors are being identified. Medical disciplinary boards are connected to state medical societies and are primarily responsible for protecting patients from doctors who make mistakes, whether through incompetence or malfeasance. How effective they are depends on the time and money they invest in examining evidence presented in malpractice suits and tracking state police reports regarding drunk driving, sexual misconduct, overprescribing controlled substances, and so on. According to the Federation of State Medical Boards, disciplinary actions by medical boards have risen by 29 percent since 1994, resulting in 4,590 punitive actions in 2003.[5] Since there is general agreement that the number of bad doctors does not exceed 5 percent, the increase in punitive actions is not being interpreted to mean that more bad doctors are out there. It probably means that boards are more aggressive in their monitoring efforts. Some informed observers say that the same 5 percent are repeatedly involved in malpractice cases and that disciplinary boards should simply prohibit them from practicing.

While it is clear that malpractice insurance companies have been raising their premiums to adjust for lost income during the first few years of the twenty-first century, most observers agree that the primary reason behind the most recent malpractice crisis is the recent escalation of jury awards.[6] The median jury award in 1997 was $500,000, jumping to $1,010,858 in 2002, even though the proportion of cases won by plaintiffs, 42 percent, is about the same.[7] What is clear is that the payout level is having a major effect on the insurance premium doctors must pay. In 2002, the average annual premium in the southern part of Florida for obstetricians/gynecologists was $211,000 (the highest in the country); for surgeons, it was $124,000; and for internists, it was $56,000.[8] It is worth noting that obstetricians are at a particularly high risk of being sued. Those who monitor these things say that obstetricians are sometimes sued not because they did something wrong but because parents want to blame someone if their baby is not perfect.

The question of whether malpractice is the most effective avenue to address poor performance on the part of doctors inspires particularly heated debate. Malpractice lawyers argue that suing doctors is the best approach for protecting patients from incompetent doctors because the threat of being penalized makes them more careful. Doctors argue that lawyers are motivated to sue even when there is no evidence of error because they stand to collect one-third of the settlement if they go to court and win or one-fourth if the case is settled out of court. Because going to court is costly whether the suit is justifiable or not, insurance companies are willing to settle out of court even when there is no evidence of medical error. This, in turn, raises malpractice premium costs for other doctors in the insurance pool and leaves an undeserved blemish on doctors' records whose cases were settled without any effort to check to see whether the claims had any validity to them. Some doctors have countersued and won. However, that takes more time, effort, and money than most want to expend.

The AMA position is that the best way to address the problem is through "tort reform." That means putting a cap on the "pain and suffering" portion of the jury award. The AMA does not argue that patients should not be compensated for lost income and future medical care costs. It argues that there should be $250,000 limit on the pain-and-suffering part of the award. As you might imagine, trial lawyers are opposed to any cap on monetary awards as are many legislators and many members of the public. There are, however, enough legislators on the other side who support tort reform to persuade a growing number of state legislatures to cap pain and suffering awards at $250,000. Tort reform was debated in Congress but failed to pass in 2003; it is likely to be reintroduced.

There are some who believe that the solution to the problem of imperfect medical results is better education. Perhaps the medical education system is the place to address reasons behind the high rate of malpractice suits in this country.

THE MEDICAL EDUCATION SYSTEM

Before the 1880s, not only could people hang out a shingle announcing their occupation, but they didn't even have to account for their training or experience. True, those who could choose the "best" (at least what was thought to be the best at the time) did ask about educational qualifications and knew how to interpret them—not that this necessarily resulted in better outcomes. In short, getting better results was tricky and unpredictable. This state of affairs permitted a range of medical training arrangements, including apprenticeships with no course work, no books, and no labs. Clearly, this was not the best way to learn about the practice of medicine. The "medical establishment" (code for organized medicine, or the AMA and its affiliates, the state and local medical societies) had been aware of this situation ever since the mid-nineteenth century. However, the people who ran these inferior schools were colleagues and fellow AMA members. The issue was a delicate one. Most doctors were not making a great deal of money treating patients, especially in communities that were not wealthy (remember, there were no insurance companies that would guarantee payment in those days). Training fees were an important source of income. Telling colleagues that they would no longer be allowed to accept such fees because the schools they were operating were inferior was not a topic that other doctors wanted to broach.[9]

The situation got so bad that by the beginning of the twentieth century the AMA decided that it had to establish some sort of evaluation system. Remember, this was happening, in part, because the knowledge base was becoming more scientific and respectable but also because training arrangements were not adequate. The AMA launched a review of medical schools, which it did not publicize, that revealed that things were even worse than what those most closely connected to the medical establishment had suspected.

The situation was resolved without much input from the majority of people in society. The elite members of the AMA shared their concerns with others in their social circle, confident that such information would not be passed on to the wrong people (i.e., the public). This is when the Carnegie Foundation became interested in the problem. The Carnegie Foundation was (and still is) devoted to improving education at all levels. In 1907, it took on the task of improving the quality of medical education. The person who was invited to assume responsibility for this assignment was Abraham Flexner.

Flexner visited all 186 medical schools and training programs in existence at the time with the aim of rating them. He was welcomed because the Carnegie Foundation was known to distribute funds to schools. It was not until 1910, just before the Flexner report was due to be released, that it became clear what Flexner was doing.[10] He graded all the schools he visited on a scale of A through F. The schools to which he had given an F packed up and closed down even before the report was out. Others began upgrading immediately. Many could not survive. By 1920, there were eighty medical schools left.

The standard against which Flexner rated all other schools was the Johns Hopkins Medical School. What is significant about using Johns Hopkins as a model is that it grounded its coursework in a scientific body of knowledge and course work rather than practical experience gained through apprenticeship. That meant two years of basic science courses before the school allowed students to see a patient under the supervision of a senior doctor. That proposition is obviously more expensive than one based on students going directly into apprenticeships. It is easy to see why Johns Hopkins was not the first choice for those with limited resources.

The Flexner report had a number of effects. It eliminated the worst medical schools, which were also the schools that prospective medical students from poor families could afford. That had an effect on the composition of the occupation. For one, it affected the chances of minority students being able to get a medical education. Two, it affected women's medical schools, which lacked resources needed to upgrade. Few women were seeking a medical education in those days, and those who did generally did not come from wealthy families. It also became more science based. The smaller number of schools meant that fewer students could be accepted, which in turn meant that the schools could be more selective. The schools could accept only the most highly qualified applicants, who were, of course, white, male, and of a higher social class.

The quality of medical education is no longer a matter of major concern. There is always some debate about whether the curriculum should include more social science to improve doctors' sensitivity to a range of issues, such as cultural differences, risky behaviors, and death and dying, to name a few. Of greater concern, at least to those who are most closely connected to the medical profession, is the cost of education. In 2003, the median student debt for medical school graduates was $100,000 from public schools and $135,000 from private schools.[11] This is worth keeping in mind when we consider how much money doctors are making.

MEDICAL EDUCATION AND THE MEDICAL MODEL

The Flexner report clearly put the medical education system on a foundation that valued science over other scholarly pursuits. This is when the "medical model" perspective on disease took hold in medical schools, and from there it took hold in the minds of the doctors as they were being trained. This goes far in explaining why doctors are not responsive to patients' complaints that do not fit into a recognizable disease pattern. If a patient's complaint cannot be verified through observable indicators and symptoms, then the problem cannot be identified, nor can it be treated using a scientific knowledge base. Physicians consider this to be obvious. Doctors do not deny the sincerity of their patients when they say that they do not feel well. The doctors' response, however, is that their patients' reports of symptoms, exclusive of any objective data, falls outside the province of scientific medical practice. Critics of the medical model point out that there are other important dimensions to being sick. After all, a person might have a fatal disease and not know it, or other people may know how sick they are but choose to work and fulfill other responsibilities as if they were in excellent health. And then there are people who feel tired, headachy, and nauseous who test out as perfectly healthy. The question then becomes, Who is sick in such cases and who is not? Doctors say they need objective proof of the presence of illness and disease in the form of indicators signaling some abnormality.

Whether we agree with their assessment or not, doctors decide who is and who is not sick. This matters more than it might at first appear. Sick-day policies at the workplace depend on it. Whether students are allowed to take makeup exams often depends on such information. In general, a doctor's diagnosis pretty much determines whether one gets sympathy for being sick or whether one is treated as a whiner. Having no good alternative, most people end up relying on doctors to say whether someone is sick or not. If a person can present a label assigned by a doctor, then that person is much more likely to be treated as if he or she is really sick and deserves to be excused for not meeting normal deadlines and responsibilities. In short, doctors have a great deal of power in designating socially acceptable labels. The question this raises is, Is this power more beneficial or more harmful to us as patients and to society as a whole? Logic requires that critics offer an alternative. That's where things fall apart. There does not seem to be much consensus regarding the answer to that question other than saying that there are other dimensions to being sick than the ones that doctors can objectively identify and that an individual's sense of those dimensions should count for more than it does.

DOCTORS AND THE ISSUE OF MONEY

Given all the complaints about doctors, why is it that we as a society are willing to pay them so much money? Getting to the heart of the matter, this is where we finally confront the idea that doctors go into medicine because of the money.

We can start by looking at the how much they earn. But first, to get a more detailed picture, let's look at the earnings of a selected category of specialists. Table 5.1 shows the median net income as well as total practice revenue for 2002.

These are median incomes (i.e., the halfway point between the lowest and the highest levels of income), which means that some doctors earn a great

Table 5.1. Physicians' Earnings for 2002

	Net income[a]	Practice revenue[b]
Pediatricians	$130,000	$350,000
Family practitioners	150,000	350,000
Internists	150,000	318,600
Obstetricians/gynecologists	220,000	500,000
General surgeons	230,000	407,000
Cardiologists (noninvasive)	250,000	500,000
Orthopedic surgeons	300,000	700,000
Gastroenterologists	300,000	550,000
Cardiologists (invasive)	360,000	780,000

Source: Wayne Guglielmo, "Physicians' Earnings," *Medical Economics*, September 19, 2003.
[a]Take-home pay.
[b]Gross income or take-home pay plus practice expenses.

deal less and others a great deal more. The fact that there is so much variation in earnings makes it harder to lump all doctors into one income category. True, they all earn a substantial amount of money. But, wouldn't you agree that there is A LOT OF MONEY and then there is A LOT OF MONEY? To illustrate, in 2002, 46 percent of invasive cardiologists (they do the diagnostic tests to determine whether cardiac surgery is indicated) earned over $400,000, but only 3 percent of family practitioners earned that much.[12] That doctors' net income is so much lower than their practice revenue is due in part to the malpractice premiums they must pay plus a long list of practice costs, including staff salaries, the costs of equipment and supplies, and so forth. But that still leaves the question of how they get paid and who decides how much they are paid.

Historically, patients paid their doctors directly for services received. Then the insurance companies came into the picture and started setting standardized fees. For the first seven decades or so of the twentieth century, only a small proportion of doctors received a salary. Those who did included medical school professors, doctors employed by government-run organizations (e.g., a county hospital, prison, mental institution), and a small number of doctors working in corporate settings such as the steel industry or an insurance company. However, most were in private practice, also called fee-for-service practice. Things have changed. The majority of doctors in private practice enter into contracts with insurance plans or organizations agreeing to accept the fees the organization pays or a certain amount of money for treating a predetermined number of patients (this is called *capitation*). Furthermore, most physicians just beginning to practice now accept salaried positions. In other words, doctors have less to say about the prices of the health care services they provide than ever before.

There's more to the matter of how much doctors can charge for their services. The fees that doctors receive are largely set by the government, specifically by the Centers for Medicare and Medicaid Services. Even though Medicare is a program that is basically for persons who are over sixty-five, the government spends so much on Medicare that it has reason to be interested in establishing controls over the monies it pays out to doctors. It has been tightening up its system of payments for the last couple of decades. In 1992 it established something called the resource-based relative value scale (RBRVS) schedule of fees. Actually, a team of economists from Harvard University worked it out in consultation with doctors and a variety of interested parties over a four-year period. There were no surprises when it went into effect. The RBRVS schedule calculated a fee for every procedure that doctors perform. By contrast, the states set the fees for Medicaid (the government plan that pays for health care services for poor people). Historically, Medicaid fees amounted to about 60 percent of Medicare fees but have risen over the past few years. In 2003, Medicaid fees stood at 69 percent of Medicare fees.[13]

Because the RBRVS schedule is so comprehensive, private insurance companies adopted it. In short, doctors have very little to say about what they can charge; that decision is being made for them. This is not to say that doctors are rolling over and playing dead when it comes to the fee schedule. They are very attentive to government attempts to reduce the fees for particular procedures and redistribute funds going to different specialties.

Social psychologists have devoted quite a bit of effort to figuring out what accounts for specialty choice. Their answers are more complex and, in my view, more convincing than the view that doctors always go where they can get the biggest bucks.[14] For instance, at some point, medical students may become impressed with the intellectual challenge offered by specialties such as internal medicine and pediatrics, which are primarily involved in diagnosing the presence of disease.[15] They may wish to have more personal contact with a range of problems and patients, which would lead them into family practice. Or, they may find that dealing with the problems of the chronically ill, elderly, or dying patients is just too discouraging and thus choose to go into pediatrics. In addition, medical students are closely observed over all those years of training and often counseled into specialties that senior faculty think are suitable for them. This means that those medical students who start out wanting to enter into the highest-paid specialties may not end up there. For example, they might not have the manual skill or the stamina to stand through hours of surgery or the personality characteristics required to make quick and irreversible judgments about the need for surgery. In short, even if one were going for the big bucks, one's plans may not work out as intended at the beginning of the journey into medical practice.

When doctors talk about their work, especially why they choose to go into a particular kind of practice (fee-for-service, straight salary, or a percentage of the group's profit), many make clear that there are other kinds of rewards that they value more than money. They talk about the gratification that comes from being involved in long-standing relationships with their patients.

In the end, the sociological message here is that doctors are shaped by the structures that operate in the health care sector. Who shapes the structures and how that happens is more controversial. That is where one's preference for one theoretical perspective or the other comes into play. Before we try to fit one or the other theoretical framework into the occupational development of the medical profession, let's consider a few of the other occupational groups involved in health sector activities.

NURSES

Nursing is the single biggest occupational category in the health sector. There are about three times as many nurses as doctors (in 1999, there were 753,176 doctors and 2,271,300 nurses).[16] Nursing provides an interesting contrast to medicine. The history of nursing is heavily influenced by the traditions introduced by Florence Nightingale. Before her work during the Crimean War in the 1880s, nursing was not considered a respectable activity for women from good families. It was considered dirty work. Nightingale emphasized the use of skills available to every middle-class young woman—namely, cleaning wounds, changing bandages, and comforting patients. By assuring doctors that nurses were there to assist them and not get in their way, she made nursing an acceptable, suitable occupation for a young woman from a respectable family. Therein lies the problem that nursing has faced ever since.

Historically, nursing care was largely performed by women in the home for members of the family, including the extended family. It was only after nursing became an identifiable occupation during the twentieth century that nurses started to work outside the home. Those who carried out their work in the patient's home were called private duty nurses. Their duties were not strictly defined, so they ended up doing a little food preparation, a little house cleaning, maybe a little clerical work—in other words, whatever the client wanted and the nurse was willing to do.

As hospitals became a more regular source of care during the twentieth century, nurses began doing more work in hospitals. Private duty nursing eventually became defined as less professional. After all, you really didn't have to be a nurse to manage the personal care needs of people who were not acutely ill. As hospitals began caring for more seriously ill patients, nurses needed to have more training.

Nurses' training continued to reflect the philosophy introduced by Florence Nightingale. Nursing schools were opened by hospitals providing something closer to on-the-job training than education with a theoretical base. Nursing students were expected to live in a dorm with strict rules, be chaperoned, and perform nursing tasks in the hospital under supervision for three years. Upon graduation they received a diploma and were qualified to take a state licensing exam leading to working as a registered nurse, or RN. The relationship between doctors and nurses is best captured in the fact that nurses were expected to stand up when a doctor walked into the room and not sit until the doctor permitted it.

At some point colleges began instituting bachelor's degrees in nursing. After completing four years of college and successfully passing the state licensure exam, a nursing student became an RN, just like the diploma graduate.

During the 1960s, when there was so much interest in advancing health care and increasing the pool of health personnel, two-year associate-degree nursing programs were created. The graduates of those programs also became RNs. This created a problem. There were now three different routes into nursing, based on different levels of education and experience. In other words, nursing as an occupation did not establish control over the educational system and entry into the occupation. More troubling was the fact that the content of nursing programs varied across the three entry routes, but the nurses were largely being treated the same way by hospitals, which became their primary employers no matter which program they completed.

Anytime hospitals faced a shortage of nurses in the past, hospitals did not address the problem by raising nursing salaries, as would happen in most other occupational sectors; they just recruited more student nurses into their diploma programs. Over the last few decades, most hospitals closed down their diploma programs. This has not benefited nursing as much as one might expect, because hospitals simply began training other kinds of workers and aggressively recruiting nurses from other countries.

That nursing has traditionally been a female occupation, that nurses have historically been employees rather than independent practitioners like doctors, and that their training does not take nearly as long as medical school are factors that explain nursing's occupational fate. However, the attention given over the last few years to the effect of nursing care on hospitalized patients may alter that fate. There is a body of evidence developing to indicate that more favorable nurse staff ratios, education, and experience all contribute to better patient outcomes.[17] This, with the unremitting shortage of nurses, has brought pressure to bear on legislators. In 2003, California became the first state to pass a statute requiring hospitals to maintain an eight-to-one patient-to-nursing-staff ratio. The conventional wisdom says that what happens in California predicts what will be happening in other parts of the country. That seems to be true in this case. In December of the same year, the Quality Nursing Care Act was proposed in Congress. It was not passed. It aimed to address the widespread dissatisfaction nurses feel regarding their work environment. Nurses say that they are being forced to assume an excessive workload, which poses a danger to patients, and that their complaints are being ignored. This is causing nurses to quit, which is one of the major factors responsible for the current shortage of nurses and the difficulty the occupation is having recruiting an adequate number of nursing trainees.

Nursing has sought to carve out niches in which nurses could work more independently. It created a number of "advanced practice" nursing programs, including those of nurse midwifery (delivering babies), nurse anesthetist, and nurse practitioner. All of these require training at the master's degree level. In addition, there are doctoral-level programs leading to a Ph.D. or doctorate in nursing. Nevertheless, doctors are legally authorized to diagnose, prescribe, and treat patients, while nurses are generally not allowed to do so. Some states give broader practice privileges to nurses, meaning that they permit nurse practitioners to have their own offices and their own patients; but even in those instances, doctors have final authority if questions come up.

Like nurse practitioners, certified nurse midwives are considered to be primary health care providers in certain underserved areas. In urban and suburban communities, nurse midwives work with doctors to manage normal pregnancies. Satisfaction studies regularly show that women are very satisfied with the care they receive from nurse midwives probably because nurse midwives allow them more control over the delivery process—for example, by allowing them to take more time to deliver. There is no difference in birth outcomes between deliveries managed by nurse midwives and doctors, which may be due to the fact that nurse midwives are willing to refer high-risk pregnancies to doctors. The question this kind of evidence raises is whether greater reliance on such "physician extenders" should be advocated more vigorously.

Nurses with advanced degrees who work in hospitals have managerial responsibilities in addition to patient care responsibilities. They oversee the work of licensed practical nurses (LPNs), who receive anywhere from six months to over a year of training); nurses aides, who receive a few weeks or months of training; and ward clerks, who are hired without special training to carry out the secretarial tasks for nurses in a hospital.

Is the largely dependent position of nurses vis-à-vis doctors and hospitals more beneficial to society or less beneficial? Or, as a sociologist might put it, is it socially functional, or does conflict theory provide a better interpretation of their situation? We will return to that question at the end of the chapter.

THERAPISTS

A range of occupational groups fall under this designation. Two of the most commonly recognized are physical therapists and occupational therapists. Activities therapists (in music or art) work with patients who are hospitalized for longer stays. Then there are the less-well-known categories of hospital therapists, such as respiratory therapists. Not all therapists work in hospitals—for example, audiologists and speech therapists may have private offices and private practices. Additionally, there are a number of occupational groups doing psychological counseling who may be regarded as therapists or counselors. In short, therapists come to this work from wide-ranging backgrounds and with a variety of degrees.

TECHNICIANS

Technicians constitute a broad category as well. Medical technicians work in hospital or clinic laboratories. It is hard to tell technicians from technologists, who usually have more education and training than technicians do but work in the same lab doing related tasks. X-ray technicians work directly with patients and have been around for a long time. There are now technicians associated with all kinds of new diagnostic equipment whose work is similar to that of X-ray technicians—for example, sonography technicians, mammography technicians, CT technicians, nuclear medicine technicians, and so on. Many new categories came on board as hospitals created new jobs and trained people to do particular tasks. For instance, hospitals trained pharmacy technicians to count pills and bottle them, blood technicians to draw patients' blood, and so on. Hospitals can and do take particular tasks and turn them into very specific occupations, such as taking a patient's temperature, taking blood pressure, giving patients injections, and so on.

Then there are emergency medical technicians (EMTs). They attend to people in an ambulance in an emergency situation. Their objective is to stabilize the patient and get him or her to the emergency room. In some ways their work is comparable to that of physicians' assistants in the sense that they take direct responsibility for the patient under the guidance of doctors. In the case of EMTs, they are able to connect patients to equipment that is monitored by doctors in the emergency room. But it is the EMTs who administer treatment.

Physicians' assistants (PAs), who do not actually fit neatly into any one of the designations, carry out tasks assigned by a physician. Physicians have been employing increasing numbers of physicians' assistants in recent years. They have increased in number from 23,300 to 50,121 between 1993 and 2003.[18] PAs may assist in surgery, do continuing care for surgical patients, go out on home visits (in some parts of the country more than others), and so on. They differ from nurse practitioners in that PAs work under the physician's license, while nurse practitioners work under their own licenses. In other words, the physician's assistant may do brain surgery if the physician who employs him or her (more often him than her, however) is willing to accept responsibility (which is not to say that hospitals would be willing to let this happen).

ADMINISTRATORS AND OTHER ADMINISTRATIVE WORKERS

Hospital administrators generally come to this work with master's degrees in hospital administration or comparable designations. The degrees are granted by business schools, schools of public health, medical schools, and a variety of other kinds of programs. The coursework is, however, not all that different. Hospital administrators must be prepared to oversee a variety of activities and occupational groups in hospitals and all the other kinds of health care delivery settings, such as extended care facilities, outpatient facilities, managed care settings, psychiatric hospitals, and so on.

The scope of their responsibility is interesting to consider. Their authority comes from the board of directors or board of trustees, depending on whether the institution is for profit or nonprofit. They have full authority and responsibility for running the organization on a day-to-day basis. Decisions involving major changes or expenses are the province of the board, which the administrator is responsible for carrying out. There is one gray area that continues to be somewhat less than clear, although it was even less clear in the past than it is at present. That is the relationship between hospital administrators and doctors.

When the majority of doctors were in independent fee-for-service practice—that is, they had admitting privileges at hospitals but were not employees of the hospital—administrators had more difficulty persuading them to abide by any rules the administrator wanted to set down. It was a matter of delicate negotiation and verbal agreement. That has changed. Doctors now sign contracts where as much as possible is agreed on before the doctor begins his or her association with the hospital. Doctors' privileges—that is, the kinds of procedures they can perform—are spelled out in the contract. Decisions about privileges are determined by committees of doctors who have the expertise to evaluate the abilities of their colleagues. The administrator's role is to make sure the committees carry out their work well. Administrators generally do not get directly involved in areas in which technical knowledge is at issue. Still gray, but not nearly as gray as it had been.

One of the biggest responsibilities that falls to administrators is overseeing record keeping. And there are records of all kinds—the usual things such as payroll records and purchasing records, of course; more complicated matters revolve around patients' medical files, insurance records, billing records, and anything that might be required in malpractice cases. Protecting the organization from malpractice is a career in and of itself. In fact, there is a new occupational role called "risk management," which is dedicated to eliminating as many opportunities for malpractice suits as possible—from making sure the railings are sturdy enough to making sure that patients who want to discuss a problem are put in contact with the appropriate person.

The medical records department in hospitals, where medical records technicians work, has been one of the fastest-growing areas in the health sector because there is so much paperwork. And it has changed dramatically over the last few decades. Until the end of the twentieth century, medical record keeping was a matter of filing pieces of paper. Now it is a matter of keeping computerized records and worrying about a whole set of new concerns — most notably, protecting the privacy of those records.

OTHER PRACTITIONERS

There are two categories of practitioners known as "limited practice" doctors: podiatrists, who are licensed to treat the full range of foot ailments; and dentists, who treat teeth and gums. Dentists and podiatrists are licensed to perform surgery and administer medications. They are doctors. These privileges differentiate them from other practitioners who may also call themselves doctors. For example, optometrists are licensed to examine the eye and prescribe lenses, but when they detect eye disease, they must refer patients to an ophthalmologist, who is an M.D. specializing in the treatment of eye disease.

Similarly, pharmacists are licensed to dispense medications but not prescribe them, even though in many instances they know a great deal more about drug interactions than doctors do. In some hospitals, clinical pharmacists with advanced degrees go on "rounds" with medical staff to explain drug interactions to medical residents.

CONCLUSION

This has been a very brief overview of the division of labor in the health sector. The topic is too big to address more thoroughly in a book that aims to provide an overview of the whole health care delivery system. The fact that we have examined only a selected number of the occupations involved in greater detail also makes it difficult to apply a theoretical framework with any accuracy. With these reservations in mind, we still might be able to raise some interesting questions without necessarily expecting to answer them fully. Of course, even much lengthier discussions might not lead to satisfactory answers to many of the questions we might want to consider.

Do you conclude at this point in our discussion that doctors have tried to arrange things to give themselves more power, more independence, more income? Keeping in mind that we can only observe how they behave, we can certainly say that they have achieved greater control over medical work than any other health occupation, which has brought them high prestige and income. Should society set some limits on this by extending the practice rights of other occupational groups? Consider the fact that psychologists have been lobbying to gain the right to prescribe medications for patients, and as of 2004 two states have granted them this right. Is this a good thing for their patients? How about for society as a whole? Allowing other health workers to perform certain medical procedures would certainly be less expensive because their education is not as long and costly and because they work for less money. Doctors say that letting people with less training prescribe powerful drugs and do more procedures poses an unnecessary risk to patients. For their part, other health practitioners say that doctors simply want to dominate medical knowledge to maintain their power and protect their high incomes. The two positions capture the essence of the functionalist and conflict theory perspectives.

Responding to the questions raised here provides the answer to a broader set of concerns: Has the division of labor in the health care system evolved as it has because society wanted to see it evolve this way? Or did the structure of this social institution evolve the way it did irrespective of the public's preferences because doctors succeeded in capturing control over medical work, thereby increasing their earnings while making great efforts to convince us that this arrangement was really socially beneficial? As you would expect, the answer depends on whom you ask.

Doctors certainly do not think that the health care system has been developed to accommodate their preferences. If you talk to doctors who have been in practice for a long time, they will tell you how great it was to practice during the "golden age" of medicine, by which they mean the 1960s and early 1970s. They say that medicine is now being controlled by "bean counters" and clerks who are more interested in keeping costs down than helping patients get well. Indeed, one measure of how strongly they feel about the changes is that they are forming unions, which they expect will finally capture the attention of all those bean counters who they say have been ignoring doctors' views. Does this mean that doctors have been losing power and control over the system? Or does it mean that they are just saying that to lobby for even greater power—that is, projecting their "construction on reality" onto it?

Personally, I find such questions intellectually stimulating. They expand one's thinking. But what is troubling is the fact that there are practical implications involved. Policy decisions are being made based on the answers we all come up with, whether those answers are good answers or not. Recognizing that this social institution must, out of necessity, operate under the auspices of decisions and policies made by someone explains why so many people are eager to participate in the process of building, expanding, and reshaping it.

Can we see the same processes operating to expand the alternative health care industry? This is the question we take up in the next chapter.

NOTES

1. "Persons Employed in Health Service Sites: United States, Selected Years 1970–2002," *Health United States, 2003* (Washington, D.C.: U.S. Department of Health and Human Services, Public Health Service, 2003), table 98.

2. Frederic Hafferty and John McKinley, eds., *The Changing Medical Profession: An International Perspective* (New York: Oxford University Press, 1993); Frederic Wolinsky, *The Sociology of Health: Principles, Professions, and Issues*, 2nd ed. (Belmont, Calif.: Wadsworth, 1988).

3. Howard Becker, Blanche Greer, Everett Hughes, and Anselm Strauss, *Boys in White* (Chicago: University of Chicago Press, 1961); Robert Merton, George Reader, and Patricia Kendall, *The Student-Physician* (Cambridge, Mass.: Harvard University Press, 1957).

4. Linda Kohn, Hanet Corrigan, Molla Donaldson, eds., *To Err Is Human: Building a Safer Health System,* Committee on Quality of Health Care in America, Institute of Medicine (Washington, D.C.: National Academy Press, 1999).

5. Damon Adams, "More Doctors Disciplined as States Bolster Medical Boards," *American Medical News* (April 26, 2004): 1–2.

6. General Accounting Office, "Medical Malpractice Insurance: Multiple Factors Have Contributed to Premium Rate Increases," October 1, 2003, GAO-04-128T.

7. Tanya Albert, "Malpractice Plaintiffs' Wins, Awards Up Slightly," *American Medical News* (April 19, 2004): 8.

8. U.S. Department of Health and Human Services, Office of the Assistant Secretary for Planning and Evaluation, "Special Update on Medical Liability Crisis," September 25, 2002, at aspe.hhs.gov/daltcp/reports/mlupd1.htm.

9. Paul Starr, *The Social Transformation of American Medicine* (New York: Basic Books, 1982), 112–23.

10. Abraham Flexner, *Medical Education in the United States and Canada* (New York: Carnegie Foundation for the Advancement of Teaching, 1910).

11. Myrie Croasdale, "High Medical School Debt Steers Life Choices for Young Doctors," *American Medical News* (May 17, 2004): 12.

12. Wayne Guglielmo, "Physicians' Earnings," *Medical Economics Archive* (September 19, 2003).

13. Stephen Zuckerman, Joshua McFeeters, Peter Cunningham, and Len Nichols, "Changes in Medicaid Physician Fees, 1998–2003: Implications for Physician Participation," *Health Affairs* web exclusive (June 23, 2004): 374–84.

14. Forrest Collins and Robert Roessler, "Intellectual and Attitudinal Characteristics of Medical Students Selecting Family Practice," *Journal of Family Practice* 2 (1975): 431–32; Charles Schumacher, "Personal Characteristics of Students Choosing Different Types of Medical Careers," *Journal of Medical Education* 39 (1964): 278–88; George Zimny and Thomas Thale, "Specialty Choice and Attitudes toward Medical Specialists," *Social Science and Medicine* 4 (1970): 257–64.

15. Peter Weil and Mary Kay Schleiter, "National Study of Internal Medicine Manpower: VI. Factors Predicting Preferences of Residents for Careers in Primary

Care and Clinical Practice or Academic Medicine," *Annals of Internal Medicine* 94 (1981): 691–703.

16. "Active Health Personnel according to Occupation: Selected Years 1980–2000," *Health United States, 2003* (Washington, D.C.: U.S. Department of Health and Human Services, Public Health Service), table 102.

17. Linda Aiken, Sean Clarke, Robyn Cheung, Douglas Sloan, and Jeffrey Silber, "Educational Levels of Hospital Nurses and Surgical Patient Mortality," *Journal of the American Medical Association* 290 (September 24, 2003): 1617–23; Linda McGillis Hall, Diane Doran, Ross Baker, George Pink, Souraya Sidani, Linda O'Brien-Pallas, and Gail Donner, "Nurse Staffing Models as Predictors of Patient Outcomes," *Medical Care* 41 (2003): 1096–1109; Julie Sochalski, "Is More Better?" *Medical Care* 42 (February 2004): II-67–73; Jack Needleman, Peter Buerhaus, Soeren Mattke, Maureen Stewart, and Katya Zelevinsky, "Nurse-Staffing Levels and the Quality of Care in Hospitals," *New England Journal of Medicine* 346 (May 30, 2002): 1715–22; Kevin Grumback, Michael Ash, Jean Ann Seago, and Janet Coffman, "Measuring Shortages of Hospital Nurses: How Do You Know a Hospital with a Nursing Shortage When You See One?" *Medical Care Research & Review* 58 (December 2001): 387–404.

18. Damon Adams, "More Family Doctors Find PAs to Be Practice Assets," *American Medical News* (November 17, 2003): 14.

6

Alternative Medicine

We believe that the combined knowledge of old and new healing modalities is ultimately superior to a single-model approach to health and wellness.

It is our philosophy that diverse modalities such as Massage, Counseling, Reiki, Yoga, Shiatsu, Biofeedback, Chiropractic, Hypnosis, Homeopathy, Naturopathy, Cranio-Sacral Therapy, the Arts Therapies, Western Medicine and many others can work in conjunction with each other as part of unified team rather than in competition. This integrated approach will lead to safer, faster and more effective healthcare.

Peter Redmond and Eric Miller
Association for Integrative Medicine
www.integrativemedicine.org/aimright.html

"Disease claims" by makers of dietary supplements are frequently made on the Internet, despite the FDA [Federal Drug Administration] ruling that these are not permitted. These findings show that the more than 280 advisory letters sent by the FTC [Federal Trade Commission] in July of 2002 to retailers warning that their Web site claims must be supported by scientific evidence cover a small portion of possible infractions.

Catherine DeAngelis and Phil Fontanarosa,
editor and executive deputy editor, respectively
Journal of the American Medical Association
September 17, 2003

A [*Consumer Reports* magazine] investigation found that many dangerous supplements can easily be purchased in stores and online. Many of these supplements have been banned in other countries. Why can't the U.S. Food and Drug Administration ban these products now?

We found that regulatory barriers created by Congress, supplement-industry pressure, and a lack of resources at the FDA have resulted in major risks for consumers.

Consumer Reports
May 2004

People have been using folk remedies and consulting local healers since the beginning of time. No one had much reason to interfere. Eventually, however, enough people in society expressed concerns about such practices that something had to be done. People found that some healers were so incompetent or dishonest that somebody, namely the government, needed to step in to regulate who could and could not open up shop as a health practitioner. The United States began licensing persons practicing healing arts as of the 1880s. From the beginning, licenses were issued by special units within each state. The states, in consultation with the associations representing groups of health providers, outlined the standards, educational requirements, and qualifying examinations for each of the occupations designated as requiring licensure. There are two special, legally defined privileges associated with the license to practice medicine—namely, the right to prescribe controlled substances (i.e., narcotics and other addictive drugs) and the right to cut into a patient's skin. Society has generally not prevented other practitioners from practicing healing arts, whether it chose to license them or not, as long as they refrained from prescribing restricted drugs and cutting into the skin.

As you recall from the last chapter, by the turn of the twentieth century, allopathic medicine had established itself as the single form of medical practice that was truly grounded in scientific principles. It continued to gain ground while the other forms of practice lost ground. Medicine's success was due to growing evidence of its efficacy as well as mainstream medicine's lobbying efforts aimed at restricting the rights of other practitioners, whose treatments, allopathic doctors, said were ineffective at best and dangerous at worst. For years, there was relatively little social concern about all those other practitioners because, with a few exceptions, they had been fading away without any additional effort on the part of society. Over the last few decades, however, ever since people in this country started complaining that doctors were treating body parts instead of the whole patient, we have been seeing a resurgence of interest in some of those other forms of care. "Wholistic," or "holistic," medicine began capturing more attention.

Still, until the early 1990s, no one had much of an idea how much the holistic health care movement had grown and exactly how many people were actually involved in seeking "alternative" health care services. A survey, reporting data collected in 1990, was published in 1993 in the *New England*

Journal of Medicine that stated how many Americans were turning to alternative care and how much Americans were spending on that kind of care.[1] It suddenly became very clear that alternative health care was a much bigger enterprise than anyone had realized. That study received a great deal of attention because it was carried out under the auspices of highly respected authors and institutions. The lead author of the study, Dr. David Eisenberg, was the director of the Center for Alternative Medicine Research and Education at Beth Israel Deaconess Medical Center and an assistant professor of medicine at Harvard Medical School. Perhaps even more significant was the fact that he began the analysis from a position open to the possibility that alternative medicine did have something beneficial to offer. He was also teaching some alternative therapy techniques and doing research to test their effects.

The Eisenberg study revealed that about one-third of Americans were using alternative therapies and spending nearly $14 billion for such care. A number of related events took place around this time that signaled the growing importance of alternative medicine. In 1992, Congress established the Office of Alternative Medicine within the National Institutes of Health to evaluate alternative therapies. Its funding was substantially increased over the next few years, and in 1998 it was renamed the National Center for Complementary and Alternative Medicine.[2] Finally, medical schools, seventy-five at last count, began adding "complementary" medicine courses to their curriculum.[3] The new label meant that mainstream medicine was willing to reconsider its assessment of alternative therapies. Within the last few years an even newer label has come into existence—"integrative medicine." The Association for Integrative Medicine was established to achieve a number of objectives, including providing a forum for professional communication—reviewing standards of clinical practice and professional credentials—which is accomplished at conferences and online. The founders of this association assert "that the combined knowledge of old and new healing modalities is ultimately superior to a single-model approach to health and wellness."[4]

Does this mean that the concerns about alternative care have now been addressed to everyone's satisfaction? Not at all. It seems that the more people use alternative therapies, the greater the controversy becomes. The eruption of the "ephedra" (weight loss medication) scandal a few years ago serves to illustrate the point. (We will get back to the matter of why no one stopped its distribution before people suffered irreparable harm, including death.) Problems such as this are not about to go away, because the number of people using alternative medicine continues to rise. The most convincing evidence comes from the same team of researchers whose study attracted so much attention during the first half of the 1990s. The follow-up study, carried out in 1997 and published in 1998, indicated that the proportion of

Americans using alternative therapies had risen from about 34 percent to 42 percent and that total, 1997 "out of pocket" (i.e., not covered by insurance) expenditures were approximately $27 billion, which is about 45 percent more than that in 1990.[5]

These facts seem rather peculiar. If mainstream medicine really can do much more for us than ever before, why are people turning to alternative medicine? Exactly who is turning to the alternative providers—the poor and uneducated who cannot afford to see a qualified doctor? Terminally ill patients who are desperate? Or is there something about mainstream medicine that is turning off increasing numbers of patients? Is there reason to try to prevent con artists from taking advantage of people, or should we treat the decision to seek alternative care as a matter of consumer choice? This chapter addresses these questions, but first we should clarify what it is that people have in mind when they talk about alternative medicine. Although there is no generally agreed-on definition, the following three efforts to define the scope of this phenomenon should provide us with a sense of what people mean when they talk about alternative therapies.

A classification developed by librarians working in medical libraries provides us with the following categorization:

- Eastern systems of medicine—examples include acupuncture, Ayurvedic medicine, Chinese medicine, Qigong, Reiki, Shiatsu
- Western systems of alternative medicine—chiropractic medicine, homeopathic medicine, naturopathic medicine, and so on
- Herbal medicine—aromatherapy, Bach flower remedies
- Manual healing methods—acupuncture, Alexander technique, Feldenkrais method, massage therapy, polarity therapy, reflexology, Reiki, Rolfing, Shiatsu
- Mind–body methods—biofeedback, hypnosis/hypnotherapy, music therapy[6]

Eisenberg's study, which laid the foundation for research on alternative care, collected information on sixteen types of therapy: relaxation techniques, herbal medicine, massage, chiropractic, spiritual healing by others, megavitamins, self-help group, imagery, commercial diet, folk remedies, lifestyle diet, energy healing, homeopathy, hypnosis, biofeedback, and acupuncture.

A review funded by the Milbank Memorial Fund, which is a nonpartisan foundation that focuses on health policy issues, found the most popular forms of complementary and alternative treatment to be acupuncture, chiropractic, homeopathy, herbal medicine, massage, and naturopathy.[7] (The discussion to follow describing these forms of practice relies on this report.)

While some therapies (such as diet) are self-explanatory, others (such as spiritual healing) are so highly individualized that they do not lend themselves to a single definition. A number of alternative therapies do, however, have an organized approach and require the practitioners to obtain training. We will examine these latter types more closely in the following section.

CHIROPRACTIC

Chiropractic is a good place to begin discussing alternative medicine because chiropractors are now the third-largest group of practitioners, after physicians and dentists. Chiropractic was founded in 1895 by an American, Daniel Palmer, who was treating patients using a variety of approaches when he determined that disease is due to misalignment of the spinal vertebrae. Spinal manipulation became his primary method of treatment. Palmer's son, B. J. Palmer, opened the first school of chiropractic medicine and continued to promote the therapy.

As of 2004, there are eighteen American chiropractic colleges. They require sixty undergraduate credit hours and four to five years of additional training. The majority of patients who turn to chiropractors do so to relieve back pain, but chiropractors also treat other health problems. The American Chiropractic Association offers certification in radiology, neurology, behavioral health, nutrition, and occupational health, to name a few areas of advanced training. Chiropractors are licensed to practice in all fifty states. Medicare pays for spinal manipulation, as do many private insurance plans.

The fact that chiropractors are licensed by the state and receive third-party payment means that what they do has become less marginalized. A major step in that direction occurred as a result of a law suit. Until 1983, the American Medical Association (AMA) referred to chiropractors as "quacks." Chiropractors sued saying that the AMA was engaged in "restraint of trade" (i.e., trying to prevent them from making a living). They won. The AMA was restrained from making such statements. Even though the AMA no longer labels them as quacks, it has continued to assert that the treatments they provide have no scientific basis.

Why should that make a difference? If people feel better, then chiropractors are doing something beneficial for their patients, right? Yes, but should the rest of us pay (through our insurance premiums and Medicare contributions) for treatments that mainstream medicine has long argued have no proven benefit, just because it makes people feel good? The mainstream medical establishment goes further. It says that chiropractors may do more harm than good by convincing patients that they do not need to see a medical doctor for their problems, which could lead to more serious illness and even death. Some representatives of mainstream medicine also say that people who visit chiropractors are spending more money than anyone realizes, if you compare the cost of office visits to a chiropractor versus visits to an M.D., because patients have to keep going back to the chiropractor to relieve pain. Are medical doctors saying this simply to "restrain trade" (i.e., keep more patients for themselves), or are they truly concerned about patient welfare?

That question is hard to answer because no one is studying doctors' motivations. So let's focus on something for which we do have some data. Mainstream medical researchers have become interested in taking a closer look at what chiropractors do. A comparison of treatment by medical doctors and chiropractors indicates that chiropractors produce similar or slightly better results when it comes to relief of back pain.[8] Researchers have found no evidence to show that chiropractic treatment of other ailments offers any clear benefit. Nevertheless, their patients insist that they could not get along without chiropractic treatments, which helps to explain why insurance companies cover chiropractic care.

There is some reason to think that insurance companies are prepared to rethink their willingness to pay for the full range of chiropractic services. Because concern about rising health care costs has become so widespread, insurance companies and others who have reason to examine the workings of our health care delivery system have been paying a great deal more attention to the results of "outcome studies" conducted to document treatment results. Closer scrutiny of the costs as well as the benefits of chiropractic treatment is likely. Unless there is clear clinical evidence of benefit, insurance companies will be far less willing pay for chiropractic treatments simply because they make people feel better.

HOMEOPATHY

Homeopathy, founded in the early nineteenth century by a German doctor, Samuel Hahnemann, is based on two ideas: first, the law of similars, meaning that "like cures like"; second, the law of infinitesimals, meaning that less is more. Treatment involves diluting, to the maximum extent, the substance suspected of causing the disease. The homeopathic remedies that homeopaths dispense have been exempted from government regulation since 1938. Since there is no separate licensure covering homeopathic treatment, homeopaths are governed by laws that govern medical doctors. Americans spend about $165 million per year for homeopathic preparations according to the National Center for Homeopathy.

How well does homeopathy work? Clinical studies reveal that homeopathy does produce positive results. However, because the treatments are highly individualized and because patients with the same diagnosis may receive different medicines, it is difficult to identify standardized treatment patterns and test their efficacy. Some researchers argue that the success of homeopathic treatment is due to the power of a placebo effect (the sugar-pill phenomenon, meaning that people get better because they believe in the power of the medicine, not because the medicine itself is powerful).

NATUROPATHY

During the late 1890s and early twentieth century, there were at least twenty naturopathic schools in existence. By the late 1990s, only two accredited naturopathic schools remained. However, several others were in the process of establishing themselves. Also, some medical schools have been adding naturopathy to their curriculum.[9] The attraction seems to be that naturopathic practitioners emphasize prevention and treatment of disease through healthy lifestyle and control of risk factors. They promote health by stressing nutrition and focusing on forestalling the detrimental effects of degenerative disease.

Licensure is uneven. Eleven states issue licenses through special boards. Other states allow naturopaths to practice but do not license them. Two states, Tennessee and South Carolina, consider the practice of naturopathy to be illegal. This may change in response to the efforts of naturopaths in six states who have been campaigning to be permitted to perform minor surgeries, prescribe more medications, and do normal baby deliveries.

ACUPUNCTURE

Acupuncture has been used in China for more than two thousand years. The technique was not well known in the United States until 1971 when James Reston, a *New York Times* columnist, reported that he benefited from it after having surgery.

The treatment consists of applying fine needles at particular points in the body. The theory behind the treatment is that life energy flows along pathways called *meridians*, which connect with internal organs. The application of needles redirects and corrects the flow of energy. In China acupuncture is used to treat many conditions. In the United States it is usually used to relieve pain. However, there is clinical evidence that it helps to address such wide-ranging problems as nausea and vomiting that accompany pregnancy, sea sickness, withdrawal from substance abuse, sinus problems, and migraine headaches, to name a few. In fact, in 1997 the National Institutes of Health, during one of its periodic conferences of experts, concluded that acupuncture is as effective as conventional medicine in some cases. It advocated further studies.

Thirty-two states regulate acupuncture. It is used by several kinds of practitioners: acupuncturists, of whom there are about sixty-five hundred, and naturopathic and chiropractic practitioners. It is estimated that approximately three thousand allopathic physicians are applying the treatment in practice. There are more than forty schools and colleges of acupuncture in the United States. Twenty of these are either approved or currently being reviewed for approval by the National Accreditation Commission for Colleges of Acupuncture and Oriental Medicine.

OTHER THERAPIES

According to the researchers who first reported on the use of alternative therapies in the United States, the three most popular therapies are relaxation techniques, herbal medicine, and massage. The role that practitioners play varies in the application of these therapies. One must learn relaxation techniques from a practitioner but may later choose to practice the techniques independently or in a group setting. Massage therapists may subscribe to an alternative medicine framework but, again, may simply offer massage without any particular theoretical backdrop.

Information on the use of herbal medicines is even harder to pin down. Patients can medicate themselves with herbal preparations either alone or in conjunction with treatment by a practitioner who is identified with a particular form of alternative practice and everything in between. This means that one can read about herbal medicine, attend lectures on the subject, share information informally with friends, rely on the advice of persons in the store where one buys the herbal remedies, or obtain information on the many Internet sites or chat rooms dedicated to this type of information.

WHO USES ALTERNATIVE THERAPIES AND WHY?

Given that in the 1997 study Eisenberg and his colleagues found 42 percent of us utilizing some form of alternative therapy, we should not be surprised to find that those who choose to use such therapies are not fringe members of society but rather your average general population of Americans. The results of the study were as follows. Females exhibited a slightly higher utilization rate than males. People aged thirty-five to forty-nine reported higher use than younger or older persons. Those with some college were more likely to use alternative care (50.6 percent) than those with no college (36.4 percent). People with an income over $50,000 (48.1 percent) had a higher rate than people with lower incomes (42.1 percent). Finally, use among African Americans was lower (33.1 percent) than that among other racial groups (44.5 percent).

The fact that lower-income people did not use alternative care as much as those with higher incomes may be explained by the fact that many of these therapies are not covered by insurance and must be paid out of pocket. The estimated out-of-pocket expenditure for alternative care in 1997 is somewhere between $27 billion and $34.4 billion. That includes $12.2 billion that went to alternative practitioners; $5.1 billion for herbal therapies; $1.7 billion for diet products; $3.3 billion for megavitamins; and $4.7 billion for books, classes, and equipment. The total amount is about the same as what Americans spent out of pocket to see their medical doctors.

So what does this tell us? If people are spending their own money and if they feel as if alternative medicine is doing them some good, what's the problem? One big problem from the perspective of mainstream doctors is concern about whether patients tell their medical doctors that they are using herbal medications. This is a major issue because there could be a drug interaction that the medical doctors need to take into account when prescribing prescription drugs and watching for side effects.

Drug interaction effects are a distinct possibility since 96 percent of the persons in the 1997 study reported that they were seeing a medical doctor at the same time that they were using alternative forms of care. However, only about 39 percent of them told their physicians about the alternative therapies. According to the editors of the *New England Journal of Medicine*, witholding information poses a number of additional potential problems that have not been given sufficient attention to date.[10] They point out that herbal remedies are not regulated, which means that the quality of the product is uncertain. There are no requirements for listing exactly what is in the product, nor is there a requirement for specifying the strength of the active ingredient. As a result, people may be taking toxic doses in the belief that taking more of these "natural" products is better. Since there is little control over production of the preparations, they may be contaminated. People may be ingesting active ingredients that they would not take if they knew about them.

This may change. In July 2003, the Bureau of Consumer Protection charged the representatives of three dietary supplement companies with fraud for claiming that one of their products, ephedra, could be used for weight loss with no risk of side effects. In December 2003, the Federal Drug Administration prohibited ephedra, its decision based on an extensive report outlining adverse effects, including heart attacks, strokes, psychiatric events, even death. In May 2004, *Consumer Reports* reported that it had examined a range of alternative medicines, concluding that twelve other supplements, in addition to ephedra, should be banned. Then there is the battle over anabolic steroids, which has been going on for some time and has not been settled as of this writing. While steroids have been prohibited by major sports organizations both nationally and internationally, steroids are widely available. That legislation introduced by Senators Joseph Biden and Orrin Hatch in October 2003 aimed at prohibiting the marketing of steroids as dietary supplements is being supported by a number of supplement-manufacturing associations suggests that greater control over dietary supplements is likely to be legislated in the not-too-distant future.

Why people take steroids is obvious—to build muscle. Why people take any of the other supplements, given the risks, is less clear. One researcher set out to find which of the prevailing explanations makes most sense.[11] The three potential explanations he examined were

1. dissatisfaction with conventional medicine because it is ineffective, has produced adverse effects, is impersonal, is too technologically oriented, or is too costly;
2. the need for greater personal control over one's body and one's health; and
3. philosophical congruence, meaning that alternative therapies are more consistent with the patient's values.

While the persons using alternative therapies in this study were of above-average education, like the people in the Eisenberg studies, in this case they were also more likely to have particular kinds of health problems, often intractable problems such as anxiety and back pain. The researcher stated that the third explanation provided the most powerful answer. He found that utilizers were more likely to have greater commitment to value systems involving environmentalism, feminism, spirituality, and personal growth psychology. The use of alternative therapies was congruent with their philosophical orientations and the meanings they attached to health and illness.

The researcher concluded that the people who use alternative therapies do not necessarily reject the kind of medicine that is conventionally practiced in the United States. They are, however, more likely to be critical of it. They generally take the position that conventional medicine in this country is too dependent on chemicals, too technological and lacking in personal touch, too restrictive in focusing on the body and ignoring the whole person. In short, a substantial number of Americans are apparently turning to health care practices that are more traditional and less dependent on Western biomedicine, or what I have referred to as the "medical model."

It is interesting to examine more closely what the traditional systems offer that is so different from conventional Western medicine.[12] It is the focus on spirituality that seems to be the common feature, which may be described as the emphasis on a "vital life force." This is true of Chinese medicine, which is influenced by several spiritual schools—in particular, Taoism; East Indian medicine, which is known as Ayurveda and is grounded in Hinduism; and Native American medicine, which owes a great deal to respect for nature and belief in spirituality. These forms of treatment are holistic in the sense that they focus on the whole person—body, mind, and spirit—rather than on parts of the person. The aim of traditional medicine is to bring the person into better alignment with the totality of his or her environment.

It is not surprising to hear that people in less-developed countries rely on many different kinds of folk medicines and rituals. Americans already believe that people in less-industrialized countries espouse beliefs that we typically label as primitive. Beyond that, they do not have access to sophisticated technology and cannot afford Western medicine even if they were prepared to use it. But how would you account for the fact that 49 percent of Australians say they use alternative therapies? In Finland, the rate is 33 percent; in Canada it is 15 percent; England and Denmark report increased use as well.[13] The Germans are not only fond of herbal medicines but have great faith in spas and the hydrotherapeutic treatments the spas provide. And, of course, we know that people in various parts of Asia have a long history of using a range of traditional medicines. Such high rates must mean that at least some of these people are middle class—that is, well-educated people with reasonable incomes.

CONCLUSION

If people want to spend money on alternative, or complementary, or integrative medicine, there is little social support for introducing measures that would prevent them from doing so. The question that is being raised by skeptics is, Should more of it be regulated? To make sure that what the manufacturers of the preparations are putting in the bottle is exactly what they claim is in there? To ensure that alternative medical providers are not actually harming patients by defining more precisely what the providers may and may not do and by licensing them? By providing funds to do more clinical testing to distinguish effective from ineffective therapies?

Interestingly, the alternative/complementary/integrative practitioners do not agree among themselves in their responses to these questions. Some believe that greater regulation will bring increased status for alternative medicine practitioners and respect for their treatments. Others are convinced that greater regulation will give conventional medicine a better opportunity to absorb what they have to offer and publicly discount what the medical establishment determines to be unsubstantiated after designing and carrying out its own clinical tests.

What about patients? Do they want more regulation? Obviously, they are prepared to use alternative therapies without any official sanctions. There are no known official surveys asking people how they feel about regulation, but the people I have asked say that it is precisely the "alternative" (i.e., unregulated aspect) that makes the therapies attractive and that regulating them would remove that feature. Are my respondents typical or a small and unrepresentative sample? I don't know. It appears that we will be exploring all of these questions for some time to come.

NOTES

1. David Eisenberg, Ronald Kessler, Cindy Foster, Frances Norlock, David Calkins, and Thomas Delbanco, "Unconventional Medicine in the United States," *New England Journal of Medicine* 328 (January 28, 1993): 246–52.

2. Stephanie Stapleton, "Alternative Medicine: Time to Talk," *American Medical News* (December 14, 1998): 26–27.

3. Jay Greene, "Complementary Curriculum," *American Medical News* (January 17, 2000): 7–8.

4. The Association for Integrative Medicine (www.integrativemedicine.org).

5. David Eisenberg, Roger Davis, Susan Ettner, Scott Appel, Sonja Wilkey, Maria Van Rompay, and Ronald Kessler, "Trends in Alternative Medicine Use in the United States, 1990–1997," *Journal of the American Medical Association* 280 (November 11, 1998): 1569–75.

6. Alternative/Complementary Medicine website (www.medsch.wisc.edu/chslib/hw .altmed), developed by the Health Sciences Library of the University of Wisconsin–Madison and the Health Web project. The Health Web is a cooperative project of the health sciences libraries of the Committee on Institutional Cooperation and the National Network of Libraries of Medicine Greater Midwest Region.

7. Milbank Memorial Fund, *Enhancing the Accountability of Alternative Medicine* (New York: Milbank Memorial Fund, 1998).

8. Paul Shekelle, "What Role for Chiropractic in Health Care?" *New England Journal of Medicine* 339 (October 8, 1998): 1074–75.

9. Jay Greene, "'New Kind of Doctor' Seeks Wider Roles," *American Medical News* (February 22, 1999): 1, 42.

10. Marcia Angell and Jerome Kassirer, "Alternative Medicine—The Risks of Untested and Unregulated Remedies," *New England Journal of Medicine* 339 (September 17, 1998): 839–41.

11. John Astin, "Why Patients Use Alternative Medicine," *Journal of the American Medical Association* 279 (May 20, 1998): 1548–1739.

12. Daniel Eskinazi, "Factors That Shape Alternative Medicine," *Journal of the American Medical Association* 280 (November 11, 1998): 1621–23.

13. Eisenberg and others, "Trends in Alternative Medicine."

7

Health Insurance

Like many other observers, I look at the U.S. health care system and see an administrative monstrosity, a truly bizarre mélange of thousands of payers with payment systems that differ for no socially beneficial reason, as well as a staggeringly complex public system with mind boggling administrative prices and other rules expressing distinctions that can only be regarded as weird.

Henry J. Aaron
New England Journal of Medicine
August 21, 2003

The fatal flaw in the system is that we treat health care as a commodity. . . . When health care becomes a commodity, the criterion for receiving it is ability to pay, not medical need. Private insurers and providers compete with one another to avoid getting stuck with the high-cost patients, so they can keep more of their revenues. But this game of hot potato takes a lot of oversight and paperwork. In fact, the hallmark of the system is the extent to which health funds are diverted to overhead and profits.

Marcia Angell
New York Times
October 13, 2002

Despite the insistence by some Blue Cross and Blue Shield plans that converting to shareholder-owned companies is the way to thrive, a new report says hardly any difference exists between the financial performance of for-profit and nonprofit mutual Blues, and in some respects the traditional plans are more efficient.

Robert Kazel
American Medical News
May 19, 2003

This chapter focuses on health insurance. Are you feeling your eyes glaze over already? You may be surprised to find how heated discussions about this topic can get. Insurance involves money, and people in this society have strong feelings about money, especially money that they have earned but are prevented from spending on themselves because the government is taking it and spending it (i.e., taxing us for things that are not providing us with a direct benefit right now and may never do so).

A sizable proportion of Americans are upset because they believe that the government is wasting their hard-earned money because the government is inherently wasteful and because it spends money on services for people who they are convinced do not deserve it. Health insurance falls into this category. Whether particular categories of people deserve health insurance is one of the core health care system issues that Americans have been arguing about for years. Although increasing numbers of Americans are coming to believe that everyone should have health insurance, many continue to believe that most of the uninsured find themselves in that situation because they are unemployed and probably not making much effort to get a job. This belief persists in spite of all the news stories saying that companies are reducing health benefits, that unions are striking over the reduction of health benefits and the increase in deductions from pay for health insurance, that some people are being denied health insurance coverage because of a preexisting health condition, and so forth.

The basic question is whether the government should step in to make sure everyone is insured. Where do you stand on this issue? Do you think the government should take responsibility for insuring everyone? How about people who are no longer working but who have worked all their lives and have reached retirement age? Should people who are disabled, cannot work, and therefore cannot get insurance through employment receive government-sponsored health insurance? How about poor people who do not have a job — should the rest of society assume responsibility for their health insurance?

The government does provide the elderly, the disabled, and some poor people with health insurance. That still leaves out many other categories — for example, persons who are between jobs, the self-employed, those who have not worked long enough at the company to qualify, and those who are working part-time while looking for a better job (recent college graduates, for example). Then there are the children. They cannot work. Should their health insurance and access to health care depend on whether their parents' employers provide family health insurance? Shouldn't the government do something to make sure that all these people have health insurance? In other words, do you think that the government should establish a national health insurance program for everyone so that we can all get health care when we need it? Or, do you believe that government-sponsored health insurance is actually a welfare program and that people who cannot get health insurance through their employers should either get another job or buy their own health insurance?

At some level the debate about insurance comes down to the choice between fixing current arrangements or scrapping it all and developing a new set of arrangements from scratch. To discuss this issue knowledgeably, we need to have a shared understanding of who has health insurance and how they obtained it. Our discussion begins with some basic information that may be obvious to some and startling to others. First, we must distinguish between public and private insurance programs. As was true in the case of hospitals, *public* is a code for "government sponsored and supported." *Private* is everything that is not run by the government. Private health insurance comes in two forms: private nonprofit and private for-profit. The difference between nonprofit and for-profit has to do with what happens to earnings at the end of the year. In for-profit corporations, stockholders, who have invested in the company with the expectation of making money, receive a share of the profits in the form of increased value of the stock they own and, in some cases, payouts called *dividends*. Nonprofit organizations have no investors and do not earn a "profit." If they take in more than they pay out, the organization puts the "excess" back into the organizational coffers. No one gets to keep any part of the excess as a bonus. The money is used to upgrade the organization's offerings, equipment, programs, and so forth.

Second, we need to differentiate between health insurance plans, which cover some portion of the cost of health care services if and when a person needs them (like car insurance); and plans that combine financing and delivery of health care services, which describes health maintenance organizations, or HMOs. In this chapter we will discuss insurance plans. Chapter 8 focuses on HMOs.

PRIVATE HEALTH INSURANCE

While it is true that every Congress since 1913 has taken up the question of creating a national health insurance program, there has been no agreement on a common plan, so there is no national health insurance plan in this country.

What we have are special programs for selected categories of people. There was no health insurance of any kind to speak of prior to the 1930s. The Great Depression played a role in inspiring the creation of a particular health insurance plan: Blue Cross–Blue Shield.

BLUE CROSS–BLUE SHIELD

The Blue Cross plan was developed at Baylor University in Dallas in 1929.[1] The hospital was struggling, as were all hospitals during that era, because so many patients could not pay their bills once the Depression hit. A review of the records revealed that school teachers constituted one clearly identifiable category of people defaulting on their bills. Baylor University Hospital came up with the following plan. It offered the Dallas Board of Education a plan whereby teachers would pay fifty cents a month for twenty-one days of hospital coverage per year. The plan caught on. In fact, it spread across the country. Over the following decade, other cities, in many cases whole states, established their own Blue Cross plans, which eventually spawned a Blue Shield addition and became established as Blue Cross–Blue Shield (BC–BS) plans.

The Blue Shield side of the plan evolved more slowly and was not nearly as successful as the Blue Cross side. Blue Shield was created to cover physicians' charges. However, it was more difficult to administer because there were so many doctors and so many different services that it was impossible to standardize rates. (Computers have, of course, solved that problem.) Also, there was no one to champion this cause. Doctors were not nearly as enthusiastic about instituting insurance arrangements for their services as hospitals.

The features of the Blue Cross side of the plan were considered quite creative at the time. First, it was conceived as a nonprofit plan, meaning that it was designed to cover its costs and not make a profit. Second, to cover the costs of something that is unpredictable, the idea was that everyone would pay the same amount even if they did not have occasion to use it. That was called a *community rate*. The cost for providing hospital care for everyone in the community who signed up for the plan plus administrative expenses determined the premium that the enrollees were charged for the coming year. A third characteristic of the plan was that it was created by a hospital whose primary concern was covering its costs. Accordingly, Blue Cross paid whatever the hospital charged.

The Blue Cross plan was not designed to monitor hospital costs. Critics have pointed this out, noting that the nature of the plan permitted hospitals to spend as much as they wanted because they were certain that their expenses would be covered. Blue Cross put no lid on expenditures. Defenders say, that is true, but there were important benefits in this arrangement. By shifting their costs to those who were insured, hospitals could provide care for people who could not afford to be hospitalized. *Cost shifting* became an item on the agenda of public debate during the 1980s. Critics said it was objectionable because it allowed hospitals to be irresponsible about their expenditures and was thus unfair to the individuals who were insured.

There was nothing underhanded or secret about cost shifting. This was the accustomed method used by doctors, and by hospitals to a lesser extent, before rates for health care services became standardized. Doctors charged richer patients more than they charged those who had less money. Everyone understood that this was happening. For those who could not pay cash, doctors accepted "payment in kind," such as having the house painted or a freshly butchered chicken or two instead of money. In practicing cost shifting, hospitals were just following a pattern that was already well established. (Critics point out that some patients received no care under these conditions if they could not find a doctor willing to treat them for no money. More about inability to pay for care and lack of insurance later in this chapter.)

When patterns of behavior are followed on a regular basis, sociologists say that the behavior patterns are being institutionalized. The emergence of the BC–BS plans provides a good illustration of the process through which society constructs a social institution. In that case, society registered rapid acceptance and approval of this particular social innovation, and so it was institutionalized.

There is one particularly interesting effect of the institutionalized process in this case that deserves a little more attention. Because Blue Cross would only pay for hospital care and not care in the doctor's office, doctors would routinely admit patients to the hospital for tests. Doctors would explain the Blue Cross reimbursement arrangements to patients and ask if they would agree to have the necessary tests done in the hospital. The catch was that, officially, Blue Cross would only pay for hospitalization if the patient was sick. Acknowledging this reality, doctors routinely admitted patients with a diagnosis that proved to be negative after the appropriate tests were performed.

Consider the implications of this pattern of behavior. It is less expensive to have tests done on people who walk in, have the test done, and go home. It is much more expensive to keep people in the hospital. Also, as long as the person was going to be in the hospital anyway, doctors ordered more tests to justify admitting the person in the first place. Remember that Blue Cross was in the business of reimbursing hospitals for the costs they incurred, so it had no reason to object to this pattern. The hospitals were fully aware of these practices. It was pretty obvious that there were a lot of healthy people being admitted. Doctors were doing it to save their patients money. Patients did not complain about the inconvenience because it did save them money. Both doctors and patients could convince themselves that this was a more efficient way of carrying out tests, that the tests would be more accurate because patients could be monitored before and after the tests, and so on. Eventually, however, health care costs did begin to climb, and people did start to complain about it. Now, who is to blame for letting the situation get out of hand?

OTHER HEALTH INSURANCE COMPANIES

Private for-profit insurance companies that sold life insurance were fairly well established by the 1930s. They exhibited no interest in offering health insurance until BC–BS developed its plan. The private insurance companies became interested during the early 1940s because demand for health insurance rose. That happened because wages were frozen during World War II, and one of the only things that employers could offer to attract workers who were scarce during the wartime period was better benefits, particularly health insurance. Employers discovered that health insurance was particularly attractive to workers. Consider how fast the health insurance business grew — in 1940, only 9 percent of the population had hospital insurance; by 1950 the proportion had risen to 50 percent.[2]

The privately owned insurance companies differed from the BC–BS plans in two major ways. First, they operated as profit-making rather than nonprofit enterprises. Second, they reimbursed their enrollees, rather than the hospitals, in an *indemnity* arrangement (i.e., private insurance companies reimbursed the individual and not the hospital for the costs incurred, meaning the hospital billed the patient directly). The private companies did not revise the payment schedule used by BC–BS. Like BC–BS, they simply paid hospitals whatever hospitals charged. The private companies made sure that they would make a profit by increasing the premium they charged each year. This worked until people started to complain about rising costs.

The for-profit insurance companies could have found ways to hold down costs much earlier, but no one was pressing them to do so during this era. The economy was booming, and health care costs were not rising very fast since insurance plans were far more limited than they are now and few insurance plans covered outpatient care. As the market for health insurance started to become more competitive, the privately owned insurance companies did begin competing on the basis of price. They began setting premiums based on an "experience" or "risk" rating rather than a community rating. In other words, they calculated how much particular groups of customers went to the hospital and set the rate accordingly. Furthermore, they began aggressively recruiting customers who would be less likely to run up high health care costs. This has come to be known as "cherry picking" and "cream skimming."

It obviously does not take a rocket scientist to figure out that you can attract more business by reducing the premium you charge. The for-profit insurance companies began marketing their plans to organizations employing younger and healthier workers who had safe, quiet office jobs. When this strategy was initially being developed, companies could retire their employees at the age of sixty-five (that is illegal now). Insurance companies were not concerned about signing up people who sat all day, probably smoked, and did not get any exercise, because the chances were good that they would not suffer ill health until after they retired (often very shortly after they retired), when the company was no longer insuring them. So the private companies succeeded in attracting the younger, healthier employees who were less likely to go into the hospital by charging them less than the BC–BS plans. The BC–BS plans (now more commonly referred to as the "Blues") could not do the same thing, because their legal status was that of nonprofit organizations (which meant that they did not have to pay taxes as long as they observed the conditions that made them nonprofits). Accordingly, the Blues could not tailor their rates to particular groups of people. They had to offer a community rate (the same rate for everyone), which was often higher than the experience rate or risk rate (which varies according to the characteristics of the group). Employers, who were becoming more interested in keeping their operating costs down, began turning away from the more costly BC–BS insurance.

How would you respond if you were heading up a Blues plan in your region? The only way you can compete with the private insurance companies is to employ the same business practices as they do. To offer competitive rates, you would have to turn yourself into a profit-making corporation, exactly like the private insurance companies with whom you must compete. Not only did Blues plans turn themselves in for-profit plans, they consolidated their operations through mergers, acquisitions, and joint ventures with for-profit insurers. By 1999, the number of BC–BS plans had fallen from 128 at the peak of expansion to 51.[3] The trend did not let up until the close of 2003. We will return to this matter in a later chapter.

PUBLIC HEALTH INSURANCE PROGRAMS

So far we have discussed private health insurance, regardless of whether it is offered by a nonprofit company such as BC–BS or one of the for-profit insurance companies. Let us now consider the public programs. There are three health insurance programs sponsored by the government: Medicare, Medicaid, and the State Children's Health Insurance Program. Before these programs were enacted, the government provided health care for members of the armed services and veterans. Some state and local government agencies across the country had developed health care facilities to treat the poor, but there was nothing systematic about such health care arrangements from place to place.

Medicare

The Medicare program was legislated in 1965 as an amendment (Title 18) to the Social Security Act (which was enacted in 1933). It went into operation in July 1966; the first full year of operation was 1967. It was designed to provide health insurance for people over the age of sixty-five. In the early 1960s, older Americans were found to be disproportionately poor and unable to buy their own health insurance after retirement. (Compared to persons between twenty-five and fifty-four, 13 percent of whom were poor, 47 percent of those over sixty-five were poor.)[4] Even if they could afford it, it was not readily available because insurance companies were not interested in offering it to individuals.

The primary criterion for Medicare eligibility is age. Most Americans become eligible once they reach the age of sixty-five. People who did not pay into social security during their working lives are not eligible. Some categories of younger persons who are permanently disabled or blind may qualify as well. Persons with end-stage renal disease (meaning it is fatal unless the person has a kidney transplant) were included in 1972 because someone in Congress advocated for it, and no one particularly objected. However, this disease category is the only exception; no other disease categories are included.

The plan is complicated. It was established as a two-part program: Part A is the hospital insurance portion, and Part B covers physicians' fees. Two newer parts, labeled Parts C and D, have been added in recent years. The option that allows people to join Medicare-approved alternative plans is sometimes called Part C, and the prescription drug plan legislated in 2003 is called Part D. Anyone who receives social security or Railroad Retirement Board benefits is automatically eligible for Part A, which is free to everyone who signs up. Part B covers doctors' services, is voluntary, and carries a monthly charge ($78.20 in 2005). The monthly premium for Part B is automatically deducted from the monthly Social Security check.

The government outlines the Medicare plan in a manual that is updated every year and sent out to all enrollees. Part A operates as follows: enrollees must pay coinsurance for each hospitalization during each "spell of illness." In 2004, this amounted to a total of $876 for a hospital stay of 1 to 60 days; $219 per day for days 61 to 90; $438 per day for days 91 to 150; all costs for each day beyond 150. There is a lifetime reserve of 60 days. Medicare pays all costs for each reserve day, but once one of these days is used, it becomes permanently unavailable for future use.

Part A also covers skilled nursing home care but sets strict limitations. Coverage is available for 100 days but only if the person is admitted after 3 or more days of hospitalization. There is no coinsurance for the first 20 days. As of the 21st day, there is a charge of up to $105 per day. After 100 days, Medicare pays nothing. Home health care and hospice care are also covered, again under strict limitations.

For Part B, which is the portion that covers the costs of care by a doctor, enrollees pay the monthly premium, a deductible of $100 once per calendar year, and 20 percent of all Medicare-approved doctor and outpatient charges. Part B also covers durable medical equipment (e.g., rental of a hospital-type bed) and certain nondurables (e.g., dialysis supplies). Laboratory tests are usually fully covered. The Medicare plan does not cover a number of things that you might expect it to cover, such as long-term nursing home care. Remember, it covers nursing home care only for those patients who have been admitted to a hospital first and only for a limited period of time. (There are a lot of people in nursing homes, so who is paying for their care? We will get to that shortly.) Medicare also does not pay for dental care, hearing aids and hearing exams, routine eye care and most eyeglasses, or such necessities as adult diapers.

Because coinsurance and deductibles can run into a lot of money, Medigap insurance has come into existence. There are ten standardized Medigap plans, which may be sold by private insurance companies as long as the plans cover whatever is specified in each plan, as identified by the letters A through J. The government publishes a booklet outlining what is covered by each of the plans. Companies are permitted to set the prices they charge and claim that they provide better administrative services. They cannot claim that they will provide more health care services than each plan specifies. That certainly makes it easier for Medicare enrollees to determine which Medigap policy to buy based on what they can afford and what they want covered. There is far less chance of confusion about what is covered because the government has eliminated what we think of as the "fine print."

What some people refer to as Part C and what the government refers to as Medicare + Choice (Medicare plus Choice) was introduced in 1997. Under this arrangement, Medicare pays private insurance companies a fixed fee to provide health care services to Medicare-eligible enrollees who choose this alternative. In some cases insurance companies offer more comprehensive coverage, including drug benefits, in return for an additional monthly premium. The number of plans grew to 345 by the following year, then suddenly declined when the government reduced the fee it paid the plans. The number of plans dropped to 145 as of 2004.[5] Approximately 11 percent of Medicare enrollees are currently enrolled in Medicare + Choice plans. Enrollment was higher before 1998, at 17 percent, when there were more plans to choose from and they were less expensive than traditional Medicare. Fewer enrollees opted for this alternative once "out of pocket" costs started to rise, from $429 per year in 1999 to $1,260 per year in 2003.

Things may change in response to new legislation. Accordingly to analysis by the Commonwealth Fund, Medicare + Choice (renamed Medicare Advantage in conjunction with the passage of the Medicare Prescription Drug, Improvement, and Modernization Act in December 2003), the government will pay insurance companies 8.4 percent more per Medicare + Choice enrollee than for enrollees in the original plan. Proponents presented it as a cost-containment measure. If you cannot figure out how it will save money, you are certainly not alone. It is hard to see how paying insurance companies more money to enroll more people to save money will reduce costs, but there are those in Congress who firmly believe that competition among Medicare + Choice plans will accomplish that. We will return to this topic in later chapters.

That brings us to the prescription drug legislation—the Medicare Prescription Drug, Improvement, and Modernization Act, or Part D of Medicare—signed into law in 2003 at the cost of $395 billion. Two months later, the White House announced that it had recalculated that figure and found that it would actually cost $534 billion.[6] The estimate was updated again in February, 2005 to $720 billion. Unfortunately this came at a time when the costs of the war in Iraq were running higher than predicted and the economy was not improving as fast as the White House had said it would. Thus, what troubles policy makers the most is the question of how we will pay for this bill. We will discuss costs in general and the prescription drug benefit in particular in greater detail in chapters 9 and 11.

The Medicare program with all of its complications is administered by an agency of the federal government, the Centers for Medicare and Medicaid Services (CMS; previously known as the Health Care Financing Administration), which enters into contracts with *carriers.* That is what health insurance companies (both nonprofit and for profit) are called when they agree to "carry out" the day-to-day administration of the program and earn a profit for doing so. The insurance companies do the paperwork and pay the bills submitted by hospitals and doctors who provide the health care services.

CMS also monitors the quality of the care it pays for. It requires that hospitals be accredited by the Joint Commission on Accreditation of Healthcare Organizations (JCAHO), which as you will recall is the organization that reviews the performance of hospitals in the United States. CMS does its own reviews as well. It monitors doctors' performance by contracting with peer review organizations (PROs). Peer review is carried out by other doctors. The idea here is that you need to be a doctor to evaluate whether other doctors are doing a good job. PROs employ a staff of workers, usually nurses, who review Medicare files for the purpose of finding unusual patterns of treatment or charges. When there is some question about treatment, doctors who work with the PRO become involved.

Now that you see how the Medicare program is set up, the question that you might want to ask is, How well is it working? The answer depends on what you want the program to accomplish. Obviously, Medicare cannot keep people from dying, nor can it keep people from aging and developing chronic illnesses. Most analysts agree that the Medicare program plays a major role in extending and improving the lives of enrollees. The next question that keeps coming up is, Could all this be accomplished at a lower cost? Here are some numbers to consider. In 1970 Medicare expenditures amounted to $7.5 billion; as of 2001, that figure stood at $244.8 billion.[7] Part of the increase can be explained by the increase in the number of people being covered, from 19.5 million to 37.6 million. Inflation is another part of the explanation. However, any way you look at it, inflated dollars or not, the amount of money involved is staggering.

Some people, mainly politicians and policy makers, warn us that the amount of money being taken out of our paychecks to pay for Medicare will not be enough to cover Medicare expenditures and that something must be done about it. Part A of the plan is funded through a 1.45 percent deduction from an employee's paycheck and the same amount on the part of the employer. Those funds go into a trust fund. Before the Medicare Prescription Drug, Improvement, and Modernization Act of 2003 was enacted, the trust fund was projected to run out in 2026. The new projection is that it will run out in 2019 because money to fund Medicare Advantage is coming out of the Part A trust fund.[8] There is no concern about Part B because the monthly premiums that enrollees pay are automatically adjusted each year. Funding is a pretty technical issue that we will not address here. However, it is a significant one and one that will not go away, especially in light of the fact that an especially big wave of people, the baby boomers, are about to get there. (Consider these two facts: about seventy-six million people were born between 1946 and 1964; the fastest growing age group in the population is the over-eighty-five group.)[9]

Medicaid

The other major public program, Medicaid, was legislated at the same time as Medicare as an amendment (Title 19) to the Social Security Act. Its first full year of operation was also 1967. Medicaid was established to provide health care services for certain groups of low-income people. They can be grouped into three categories: the poor elderly, people with disabilities who are too disabled to work, and poor people (generally women with small children). Adults with no children who are not disabled have not been eligible in the past. That has changed in some states. Each state determines who is eligible and how poor a person has to be to qualify. According to the federal government, the poverty guidelines for 2004 set the cutoff for a single person at $9,310 and a family of four at $18,850. However, the Medicaid cutoff has been as low as 24 percent of poverty in some states in past years. Clearly, Medicaid was not designed to cover all, even most, poor people.

Medicaid is a joint federal–state program. The federal government picks up half of each state's Medicaid outlay, more if the state has an especially high proportion of poor people. This averages out to 57 percent. The federal government allowed states a fair amount of leeway in determining eligibility, but Congress has periodically enacted new requirements linked to expanded federal support. As of 2003, Medicaid legislation now mandates eligibility for twenty-eight categories of people and allows states to cover up to twenty-one optional eligibility groups.[10] For this reason, the numbers and categories of people enrolled in the Medicaid program have been growing. Consider the trends, as presented in tables 7.1 and 7.2.

The recipients—that is, the enrollees—do not necessarily seek health care. So it is important to look at who the beneficiaries are—that is, those who are utilizing Medicaid services.

In discussing quantitative material such as this, it is always best to start analyzing tables by identifying the "biggest" facts. In this case, the biggest facts are that enrollment in the Medicaid program has more than doubled over the last twenty years, that the amount of money involved is now about twenty-eight times greater, and that it is now the biggest publicly supported health plan in the country. What explains that? Look at who falls into the largest group of enrollees. It is children. Now look at who makes up the largest category of beneficiaries. Far more is spent on the blind and disabled plus the aged than on children. That is not hard to understand. Children, even poor children who may not have the best diets and living conditions, are likely to require less expensive care than those who are chronically ill, which is more likely to be true of disabled and aged persons.

Table 7.1. U.S. Medicaid Enrollees, 1972 and 2000

	1972[a]	*2000*
All recipients	17.6M	42.8M
Aged (65 and over)	18.8%	8.7%
Blind and disabled	9.8	16.5
Adults in families with dependent children[b]	17.8	20.5
Children under age 21	44.5	46.1
Other[c]	9.0	8.6
Total	*100%*	*100%*

Source: "Medicaid Recipients and Medical Vendor Payments, according to Basis of Eligibility, and Race and Ethnicity: United States, Selected Fiscal Years 1972–2000," *Health United States, 2003* (Washington, D.C.: U.S. Department of Health and Human Services, Public Health Service, 2003), table 137.

Note: Percentages may not add up due to rounding.

[a]The year 1972 is used instead of 1967 because this is the year when the government began calculating the categories of people who receive benefits in contrast to those who are enrolled.

[b]Formerly, persons who qualified for Aid to Families with Dependent Children (AFDC), which was abolished and replaced with the Temporary Assistance to Needy Families (TANF) program in 1997.

[c]Includes persons deemed medically needy by some states. This category fell to 1.7 percent by 1995 but has obviously increased since then.

One other seemingly contradictory trend is worth noting. While the number of elderly covered by Medicaid has declined, payments for care have not declined very much at all. The decline in the number of elderly being enrolled is easy to explain. There are simply not as many poor elderly as there were in 1967, when the program was enacted. So why is nearly a third of what Medicaid spends going to cover the elderly? The answer is that the money is largely spent on nursing home care. Remember that Medicare covers nursing home care for a limited period and only after hospitalization. What about people who

Table 7.2. U.S. Medicaid Beneficiaries, 1972 and 2000

	1972	*2000*
All payments	$6.3B	$168.3B
Aged (65 and over)	30.6%	26.4%
Blind and disabled	22.2	43.2
Adults in families with dependent children	15.3	10.6
Children under age 21	18.1	15.9
Other	13.9	3.9
Total	*100%*	*100%*

Source: "Medicaid Recipients and Medical Vendor Payments, according to Basis of Eligibility, and Race and Ethnicity: United States, Selected Fiscal Years 1972–2000," *Health United States, 2003* (Washington, D.C.: U.S. Department of Health and Human Services, Public Health Service, 2003), table 137.

Note: Percentages may not add up due to rounding.

need nursing care because they are chronically ill, frail, or confused or because they need help medicating themselves, toileting, eating, and so forth? The determination that the person needs long-term nursing home care in such cases is made by the family, and a period of hospitalization is not usually involved. How does nursing home care get paid for under these circumstances? Increasingly, people who are sick enough to go into a nursing home give up whatever money they have to their children, which makes them impoverished and eligible for Medicaid. The other alternative is to pay for it out of one's own pocket. Considering that nursing home care costs at least $4,000 per month, while Medicaid coverage is free, you can understand why Medicaid has become a major alternative and is now providing coverage for an increasing number of people in nursing homes.

The disabled category has been growing because increasing numbers of people are meeting the criteria for disability. Beyond being unable to work, applicants must prove that they are poor enough. Obviously, this means that they must have incomes below whatever the state has set up as the cutoff. That is considerably more complicated than it might first appear. What if a person receives a pension the person can live on but runs up such high medical bills that he or she ends up being impoverished with very little money left to live on? This is called the *spend down* provision. A person may become eligible because so much of his or her money (e.g., social security check or pension) is going to pay for medical bills.

Consider the full implications of spending down. A person must cash in everything she owns before she can say she is truly impoverished. ("She" is appropriate here because poor women outnumber poor men: they outlive men; they bear the primary responsibility for supporting children; and they earn less so have less of a savings cushion.) That, of course, means that the person cannot own a house, a car that is worth more than whatever the state decides, and so on. Finally, the person must prove that he or she is poor. That is called the *means testing* feature of the program. Means testing is used to determine whether one is as poor as one claims to be. Accordingly, all financial records must be submitted to the state agency that carries out the review. The standard cutoff has long been $5,000 but is now $6,000 in some states, meaning that one must cash in everything that might put one's "wealth" over that line.

Critics of the Medicaid program see this as one of its most objectionable characteristics. They say that it is degrading and stigmatizing to have to prove that one is poor. There are also those who work with the Medicaid population who find no feelings of stigma on the part of Medicaid enrollees. Others object to the cost of carrying out such reviews. The administrative costs of running Medicaid are difficult to assess. However, it is not hard to see why it would be costly given how much paperwork and clerical time is involved in verifying eligibility and conducting means testing. Administrators of clinics that provide health care to the poor say that about a third of the premium such organizations receive from government programs are wasted because they are used to cover the administrative costs of reenrolling people.[11]

State Child Health Insurance Program

The State Childrens' Health Insurance Program (SCHIP or SHIP), or Title 21 of the Social Security Act, is the third major public health program. It was passed with the budget reform legislation of 1997. It was legislated in response to what we and everyone else who looks at these data have all discovered — that children, especially poor and near-poor children are at particularly high risk of being uninsured. SCHIP provides federal funds to insure children under the age of nineteen whose family income is up to 200 percent of the federal poverty level, which is higher than Medicaid in most states. Even if there is general support for providing health insurance for children, the challenge has not been easy to enroll children of families in which the adults are not poor enough to qualify for Medicaid. States use three different models for establishing and administering SCHIP: separate SCHIP program, Medicaid expansion, and some combination of these. The 2004 estimate is that 32.1 million children were eligible, but only 44 percent of them were enrolled.[12]

Congress appropriated $40 billion over ten years for SCHIP, with the provision that the states had to have administrative procedures in place and were already enrolling children. It took states longer to do this than anticipated, which meant that allocated funds were not spent. That led to new controversies. A number of states applied for such unspent funds to cover childless adults. Some policy makers objected saying that this was a distortion of the intent of the law.[13] Congress dealt with the problem of unspent funds by passing a so-called SCHIP Fix in 2003, which allowed states to get back some of remaining unspent funds. It appears that a great deal of attention is going into analyzing structure and distribution of these funds rather than measuring impact. That can be explained in part by the general agreement that SCHIP has been beneficial where it is operating effectively. The primary concern, however, is just that — getting it to operate effectively.

THE UNINSURED

According to the U.S. Census Bureau, over 15 percent of the population, or 43.6 million people under age sixty-five, had no insurance in 2003. That is how many are uninsured for the full year. If you count people who were uninsured for part of the year, then the number increases to 81.8 million to 84.8 million, which is more than a third of all Americans.[14] If you count only low-income Americans, then the figure jumps to about 70 percent.

As I said earlier, many people in this country believe that the uninsured are in that position because they are unemployed. The fact of the matter is that 78.8 percent of those who were uninsured in 2003 were employed full-time or part-time; 5.7 percent were seeking work, leaving 15.5 percent who were not in the labor force—this includes the disabled, chronically ill, and family caregivers.[15]

The ranks of the uninsured swelled in recent years as employer-sponsored health insurance began to decline. The reduction was due to the downturn in the economy that we experienced since the turn of the twenty-first century, which resulted in increased unemployment and an increase in the number of people accepting part-time and low-wage work with no health benefits. There has been a slight increase in the number of persons covered by Medicaid, but the majority of persons who found themselves unemployed did not quality for Medicaid.

You might think that some of the people who have lost their health insurance should be able to buy it on their own. There are two clear reasons to explain why they do not—one is that it would be really expensive, and two is that they may not be able to get it even if they have plenty of money to spend on it. Given that the cost of family coverage was about $9,000 and individual policies were about $3,300 in 2003 when negotiated by employers for a large group of people, the cost would be daunting on an individual basis, even for those who are well-off. More surprising to people who seek to purchase insurance on their own is finding that insurance companies can deny coverage on the basis of a person's health record and can refuse to cover anything that might lead to high health care costs.

There is legislation requiring insurance companies to provide continued coverage for a certain period after the employee leaves his or her place of employment. This is known as COBRA (passed in 1986 under the Consolidated Omnibus Budget Reconciliation Act). Since the legislation does not address the matter of costs, insurance companies can charge whatever they want for continued coverage, which a person who is now unemployed might not be able to afford. Consider the tale told by a couple in their early forties who quit their jobs to become self-employed entrepreneurs in the spring of 2004. They had this to say:

> At least we have COBRA until we straighten this out, we thought. But it's $1,300 a month! . . . That's when the sinking sensation began. . . . We had been

judged uninsurable—branded with a Scarlet U by one of the most reputable firms in the business. And the fact that we were reasonably well off financially couldn't help us fix the problem.

It was only when we got past the shock and focused on the reasons we were being denied coverage that anxiety turned to anger. . . .

Jody's Flonase? She used that nasal spray for sinus problems before flying— like a million other people. Her skin creams? They were totally cosmetic—and she paid for them herself anyway. Her neck spasm, which she woke up with one morning a few months earlier, went away with minor treatment. Most people think Jody is much younger than she is. Blue Cross made her sound as if she were falling apart.

And Matt's eyes? It was true: Matt had a weird episode three years earlier. A little wispy something in his field of vision. . . . It turned out to be tiny blood clot behind his retina, which went away by itself. He takes a baby aspirin every day as a precaution. Our doctors say it's fine. Now Blue Cross said it meant it couldn't offer him insurance. If that's the case, we thought, could it be offering insurance to anyone who is over 35?[16]

Surprising, isn't it, to discover that people who are well-off might not be able to get insurance even if they were willing to pay a fair amount of money to get it? Insurance companies are well aware of the fact that about 5 percent of enrollees run up most of the costs. Knowing this, they calculate the risks posed by the population they are selling insurance to—that is, a particular company's employees—and set the rates accordingly. Enrolling individuals is much riskier, especially individuals who have had previous health problems. Enrolling such people is a risk that just does not make sense from the perspective of insurance companies. Why accept such risk if you do not have to? And insurance companies do not have to, nor are employers obligated to offer health insurance. Unfortunately, even such draconian efforts as eliminating the highest users of health insurance has not made individual insurance more affordable or available. Those individuals who insurance companies are willing to insure on an individual basis find that the insurance available to them is generally limited and quite costly. As a result, only about 4.5 percent of the population purchased private insurance in 2001.[17]

What about companies that employ young and healthy people who are engaged in risky work—for example, logging or certain kinds of construction— or small companies that run up high costs because one or two employees experience catastrophe health problems? It means that those companies have been finding their insurance coverage becoming more expensive and in some cases unavailable. It is ironic, isn't it, that the people who need insurance the most are exactly the ones who are being pushed out of the insurance pool!

DOES INSURANCE COVERAGE MAKE ANY DIFFERENCE?

In the end, how much does it really matter whether people have insurance or not? There is a growing body of evidence to suggest that it does make a significant difference. According to the Institute of Medicine (the quasi-governmental organization created to advise the government on health issues), which brought together a panel of experts to examine the evidence regarding this question, about eighteen thousand Americans die prematurely because they do not have health care coverage.[18] Another extensive review of the literature, one sponsored by the Kaiser Commission on Medicaid and the Uninsured, found that having health insurance reduces mortality rates by 10 to 15 percent; that the uninsured are more likely to be hospitalized for an avoidable condition, which costs about $3,300 per stay; and that poor health affects educational attainment, which reduces earnings potential by 10 to 28 percent and often leads to reduced work by a family caregiver.[19]

As if being sicker and poorer was not bad enough, uninsured people find that they are charged more than those who are insured when they do go to the hospital. They have no bargaining power to negotiate over charges that large insurers can demand.

There are some people who would say that the answer to the question of health insurance coverage is obvious on the face of it. Everyone should have the same level of access to health care as a right. This is the richest country in the world and could well afford health insurance for everyone. They say that not insuring so many people is a national disgrace. Those on the other side of this debate continue to say that people should be encouraged to purchase their own insurance; then they would appreciate it more, shop for the best plan to suit their needs, and not take for granted the costs of health care as much as they do now.

HEALTH INSURANCE FROM A THEORETICAL PERSPECTIVE

Health insurance lends itself fairly well to analysis from the two theoretical frameworks outlined in chapter 2. Which do you think fits the health insurance situation better, functionalist theory or conflict theory? Remember the functionalists would argue that society has constructed this social institution the way it has because the arrangement serves society's needs. The conflict theorists would say that our health insurance arrangements permit the haves to benefit and the have-nots to get the short end of the stick, again.

Some of the fine points that come into this discussion might include the following. It is not remunerative to sell health insurance to individuals, so private insurance companies will only do so if they can charge enough to make it worthwhile. But, people who do not work full-time generally cannot pay for any insurance, let alone high-cost insurance that provides restricted coverage. So who is left to pay for it? The obvious answer is the government, which leads to a bigger set of questions and a broader range of arguments. Thus, some people say that those who do not hold down full-time jobs cause a disproportionate number of the social problems that plague society. Unemployed young men involved in gangs come immediately to mind. However, they are not the only ones. How about those who are working part-time while trying to find a full-time job? Or those who are working full-time at low-wage jobs that do not offer benefits?

Others argue that linking insurance to employment is the very heart of the problem. At this point it becomes difficult to separate the participants in this debate into two clearly identifiable theoretical factions. One of the loudest advocates of breaking the link between employment and health insurance has been that well-known member of the haves, Lee Iacocca, former CEO of Chrysler Corporation. When he was at the helm of Chrysler, he argued that providing health insurance was keeping Chrysler from being as competitive as it could have been in comparison to automobile manufacturers in other countries, where the cost of health insurance is not foisted onto the private sector. (The most recent figure I have heard mentioned is that employers are spending on average $4,400 per employee in this country.) Most fellow haves do not share Iacocca's view. They have generally opposed government-sponsored health insurance of any kind. The fact that Iacocca and a few others in his circle have been so vocal in demanding that the government take over health insurance makes identifying who the players are in this debate considerably more confusing.

Since functionalists do not generally announce themselves as such when they discuss health insurance (although representatives of the insurance industry have consistently said that things are working just fine as is), we must identify their theoretical loyalties by examining the statements they make more carefully. I should point out that there is no body of functionalist literature on health insurance, so we must look at the views being expressed and classify them as consistent with functionalist theory ourselves. Accordingly, a benevolent functionalist's view of the problem presented by health insurance might go something like this. Yes, it is clear that people should have access to health insurance because not having access makes people susceptible to more serious illness, which is more costly to society. Therefore, some policy analysts advocate letting people "buy into" Medicaid and Medicare. In other words, pay an insurance premium, possibly on a sliding scale. A less-benevolent view might be that the system is fine as it is; after all, ours is the "best system in the world," and we should not do very much to change it and jeopardize what is good about it. Minor changes and improvements are, of course, always desirable. But the only major change that this faction of functionalists would likely treat as unquestionably advantageous is anything leading to greater technological advancement.

Conflict theorists, who are more likely to state their theoretical loyalties up front, define the problem pretty much the same way but favor a different set of solutions than do the functionalists. They would prefer to dismantle Medicaid, which they say is not only demeaning but institutionalizes a two-tier system of care in which the second tier gets second-rate care. Some, but not all, conflict theorists favor moving toward a one-tier system, meaning that all Americans would have access to the same level of health care. Some groups, whose values are not neatly aligned with either of the two sociological camps—the American Nurses Association, for example—have come out in favor of extending Medicare to all Americans. The advantage would be that everyone would have to share in the implications of any reductions or improvements in services. People would be more reluctant to cut back on funding of health services if they thought this would have a negative impact on their access to health care services. A universal health care system would, of course, have to be run by the government. That quickly gets us into discussions comparing the U.S. system to those in other countries and into talk about socialized medicine. We will address this topic in chapter 10.

Before we talk about other systems, we should discuss a feature of the U.S. system that we have only touched on in this chapter, which is the growth of managed care and the subject of the next chapter.

NOTES

1. Sylvia Law, *Blue Cross—What Went Wrong?* (New Haven, Conn.: Yale University Press, 1974).

2. Rosemary Stevens, *In Sickness and in Wealth* (New York: Basic Books, 1989), 259.

3. Bruce Japsen, "Illinois Blues Balk at Go-Public Stampede," *Chicago Tribune*, June 10, 1989, business section, 1, 4.

4. Marilyn Moon, *Medicare Now and in the Future* (Washington, D.C.: Urban Institute Press, 1993), 25.

5. Henry J. Kaiser Family Foundation, "Medicare, Medicare Advantage Fact Sheet," March 2004, www.kff.org.

6. Robert Pear and Edmund Andrews, "White House Says Congressional Estimate of New Medicare Costs Was Too Low," *New York Times*, national, February 2, 2004, A14; Robert Pear, "New White House Estimate Lifts Drug Benefit Cost $720 Billion," *New York Times*, late edition, February 9, 2005, A1.

7. "Medicare Enrollees and Expenditures and Percent Distribution, according to Type of Service: United States and Other Areas, Selected Years 1970–2001," *Health United States, 2003* (Washington, D.C.: U.S. Department of Health and Human Services, Public Health Service, 2003), table 134.

8. Markian Hawryluk, "Medicare Faces Cash Crunch," *American Medical News* (April 5, 2004):

9. "Long-Term Care: Baby Boom Generation Presents Financing Challenges," testimony before the Special Committee on Aging, U.S. Senate, statement of William Scanlon, director of health financing and systems issues (Washington, D.C.: General Accounting Office, 1998), 4.

10. Lynn Etheredge and Judith Moore, "A New Medicaid Program," *Health Affairs* web exclusive (August 27, 2003): 9 pages.

11. Joel Finkelstein, "Millions Have Health Coverage Gaps—Commonwealth Fund Study," *American Medical News* (December 1, 2003): 10–11.

12. Karl Kronebusch and Brian Elbel, "Enrolling Children in Public Insurance: SCHIP, Medicaid, and State Implementation," *Journal of Health Politics, Policy, and Law* 29 (June 2004): 451–89; Karl Kronebusch and Brian Elbel, "Simplifying Children's Medicaid and SCHIP," *Health Affairs* 23 (May/June 2004): 233–46.

13. United States Government Accountability Office, "SCHIP: HHS Continues to Approve Waivers That Are Inconsistent with Program Goals," January 5, 2004, GAO-04-166R.

14. Finkelstein, "Millions Have Health Coverage Gaps," 10.

15. Families USA, "Going without Insurance" (June 2004), at www.familiesusa.org.

16. Jody Miller and Matt Miller, "Singled Out," *New York Times Magazine,* April 18, 2004, section 6, 49–50.

17. "Private Health Insurance Coverage among Persons under 65 Years of Age, according to Selected Characteristics: United States, Selected Years 1984–2001," *Health United States, 2003* (Washington, D.C.: U.S. Department of Health and Human Services, Public Health Service, 2003), table 127.

18. Michael Marmot, "Improvement of Social Environment to Improve Health," *Lancet* 351 (January 3, 1998): 57–60; Redford Williams, "Lower Socioeconomic Status and Increased Mortality," *Journal of the American Medical Association* 279 (June 3, 1999): 1745–46; Richard Wilkinson, *Unhealthy Societies* (London: Routledge, 1996); Cathy Schoen and Catherine DesRoches, "Uninsured and Unstably Insured: The Importance of Continuous Insurance Coverage," *Health Services Research* 35, part II (April 2000): 186–206; Institute of Medicine, *Care without Coverage: Too Little, Too Late* (Washington, D.C.: National Academies Press, 2002).

19. Jack Hadley, "Sicker and Poorer: The Consequences of Being Uninsured," the Cost of Not Covering the Uninsured Project, Henry J. Kaiser Family Foundation, briefing charts (May 10, 2002), www.kff.org.

8

From HMOs to Managed Care

One observer suggested that "asking PPOs [preferred provider organizations] to be more responsible for quality of care is like trying to eat soup with a fork."

> Robert E. Hurley, Bradley C. Strunk, and Justin S. White
> *Health Affairs*
> March/April, 2004

Americans rank HMOs "Dead last" among 15 national institutions in terms of confidence . . . a survey by the Gallup organization reported. . . . Women, who the survey said tend to be the key medical decision makers for families, have especially low confidence in HMOs, with just 14% expressing "a great deal" or "quite a lot" of confidence in them.

> *American Medical News*
> August 4, 2003

The term *managed care* came into common use during the 1980s. Managed care programs and structures were created for the express purpose of managing patients' care. Doctors, in consultation with their patients, had of course been managing patient care all along. According to some critics, however, there was in practice very little consultation and far too much management on the part of doctors. (Sounds like conflict theory, doesn't it? I should note that conflict theorists did not intend to have their objections to what they called "medical dominance" result in managed care; they do not like the way it turned out, which they might be labeling "managed care dominance" if the same set of critics were still doing the criticizing today.) Managed care set out to revolutionize the process through which we all receive health care services by applying practices familiar to the corporate sector—vertical integration, economies of scale, and reengineering, which translate, respectively, into buying up companies that provide the essential goods and services used by this sector; forming purchasing coalitions that can negotiate lower prices on supplies; and increasing profits by eliminating inefficiencies through centralization of administrative functions to avoid having several people doing the same job, which most people see as firing a lot of people. This moved the managed care approach to health delivery to an even newer version—managed competition (i.e., many managed care organizations competing with each other). How does all that benefit patient care? Again, to answer this question, we need to start with the basic building blocks rather than go directly to the most recent innovations in health care delivery arrangements.

Managed care was built on a network of HMOs (health maintenance organizations), which grew out of the idea that health care services should be paid for in advance. The idea of prepaid care begot HMOs, which begot managed care, which begot managed competition. Sound monumental? Actually, the story behind it all is quite simple and straightforward. The only thing that may still be confusing by the time you finish this chapter is the fact that people use the terms *HMO* and *managed care* to mean the same thing. That's not all that bad, as long as you know what the original meaning of each concept is. In fact, their ad campaigns indicate that the managed care organizations (MCOs) would prefer to be called *health plans*. (At this point, you may be ready to join critics across the political spectrum who occasionally get fed up with the labels and refer to it all as health care alphabet soup.) Indeed, the association that represents managed care organizations changed its name a few years ago to the American Association of Health Plans. Thus, you may find that the labels—HMO, managed care organization, and health plan—are now all being used interchangeably.

It seems that after some small, false starts throughout the country, the idea of prepaid care took root in 1938 with the construction of the Los Angeles aqueduct. The work was to be carried out in an area that was unsettled, meaning that living conditions were primitive. Workers were willing to tolerate that, but they were not willing to do dangerous work without some assurance of medical care. No doctor would go to such a setting without some assurances of his own, namely that he could make enough money to set up an office and meet office and living expenses. Henry Kaiser, who headed the company doing the building, hit on a solution. He would guarantee the doctor a predictable income by arranging to have his workers contribute five cents per day to assure themselves of the availability of health care services, whether they needed care or not. That worked so well that Kaiser set up similar programs for his employees during World War II to attract workers to jobs at his shipyards and steel mills in other locations on the West Coast. In 1942, he created a separate organization, Kaiser Permanente, to handle the prepaid health care arrangements for his workers.

When the war ended, wartime production declined and employment shifted to other sectors; it looked like Kaiser Permanente would not survive. Henry Kaiser saved the plan by opening it up to the public. And as they say, the rest is history. Kaiser Permanente evolved into the largest single prepaid care system in the country. By 1996, it had 6.6 million enrollees (20 percent of all Americans enrolled in prepaid care) with offices in seventeen states. Its fortunes reversed somewhat since then. In 2004, it reported serving 8.2 million people in nine states (about 11 percent).

A few other prepaid plans, which stayed local, came into existence at about the same time as the Kaiser plan. The Health Insurance Plan of Greater New York and the Group Health Cooperative of Puget Sound were two of the largest. Prepaid care arrangements were rare because there was so much opposition to them from the medical establishment (i.e., the American Medical Association [AMA] and its state and local affiliates). The fee-for-service exchange between the doctor and the patient was one of the traditional, and essential, attributes of medical professionalism according to the AMA. Accordingly, medical societies pressured hospitals to deny admitting privileges (i.e., the right to hospitalize patients) to doctors who were not in a fee-for-service practice. This forced the prepaid plans to build their own hospitals.

The plans that emerged during the first half of the twentieth century were established as nonprofit entities. The nonprofit aspect is significant. Remember, this means that there are no shareholders and no profits to distribute. If earnings exceed projected costs, the surplus (i.e., extra money) is plowed back into the organization. (As of 2004, of the ten largest managed care organizations, only the two largest BC–BS plans and Kaiser Permanente operate on a not-for-profit basis.)

The way it works is that patients and doctors must sign up with the HMO. Doctors do so by signing a contract. The earliest HMOs paid doctors a salary; others offered doctors a contract specifying a fixed amount of money per capita—a capitation fee. As managed care developed, payment arrangements became more complicated. HMOs are now more likely to use capitation plus incentives for meeting the organization's budgetary objectives. Patients sign on by enrolling in the plan. They and/or their employers agree to pay a fixed amount of money to guarantee that they will receive health care services as needed. This is called the premium. Patients must go to the doctors associated with the HMO they sign up with. Point-of-service plans (POS) evolved to allow patients to seek care from doctors outside of the plan for an extra charge each time they went out of the plan. Preferred provider organizations (PPOs), which are only slightly more expensive than HMOs, have been growing in popularity. They allow patients to select a doctor from an authorized list.

So far we have been discussing prepaid care. We still have not gotten to the story behind how HMOs and managed care came into existence. The HMO was invented in 1974—the term, not the ideas behind it. At the time, President Nixon was searching for a way to put limits on the growth of medial care costs. It had become apparent that the costs of Medicare and Medicaid (established in 1965) were running over initial cost projections. Advisors convinced President Nixon that prepaid care was the solution. Advocates argued that prepaid care would result in savings because the arrangement would encourage people to seek care earlier, before their problems became more complicated and costly to treat. So not only was it going to save money, but it would also be good for people. President Nixon presented a plan to the country that would help people maintain the citizens' health, which is where the "health maintenance" label comes from. The medical establishment could not object to this presentation, even though it was firmly opposed to the prepayment feature. The AMA labeled it "socialized medicine" in a massive media campaign. The AMA's objections not withstanding, legislation requiring employers to offer this option to their employees and funding to support start-up costs passed, and the term *health maintenance organization,* or HMO, came into widespread use.

The legislation stimulated a great deal of public interest, which eventually brought many new parties into the prepaid care business—and *business* turns out to be the right word, too. Initially, the groups that took encouragement from the HMO legislation used Kaiser Permanente as their model. They established themselves as nonprofit organizations. However, it did not take long for that to change. Within a few years, HMOs were being established with the understanding that producing a profit for their owners was exactly what the owners had in mind. Many of the new HMOs were established without enough planning, funding, or thought given to administration. Not surprisingly, many failed.

By the late 1970s HMOs were beginning to develop a bad reputation, more so in some parts of the country than in others. Some of the struggling HMOs were bought out, others simply folded up shop and disappeared. In either case, patients had to sign up with another, possibly another new and untested organization, with new doctors, different rules, and so on. This is when the idea took hold that the health care sector was inefficient, lacking in managerial talent, and backward in the application of the latest business techniques. It is also when health sector corporations became more aggressive in their efforts to operate more efficiently.

THE GROWTH OF MANAGED CARE

The corporate executives who moved into the HMO business quickly realized that one of the main obstacles they faced in trying to control costs was that the HMOs could only control the costs of patient care taking place within the doctor's office. However, once patients were admitted to the hospital, the HMO lost control. HMOs did have contracts with hospitals covering basic costs per day but could not really control the additional costs incurred once the patient was admitted. Thus, how long a patient was there, what tests were performed, how many times tests were repeated, which all have a big impact on costs, were not under the control of the HMO. The solution was to get more control over the hospital and, while they were at it, control over every other stage of care. That meant managing the care of the patient at all stages of treatment. This is what got us to the era of managed care. Managing patient care led to managing the organizations and all the personnel that patients interact with.

Regarding personnel, HMOs had traditionally relied on doctors who were generalists or primary care practitioners, as opposed to specialists or surgeons, to a greater extent than was true outside of the HMO. The internists, pediatricians, and family practitioners (the primary care practitioners) were expected to act as gatekeepers. They were, and still are, responsible for treating most of the patients' problems—referring patients to a specialist only if a problem truly required considerably more specialized knowledge. By monitoring the patients' care more closely, gatekeepers kept patients out of the hospital, which is beneficial to the patient (unless, of course, that effort becomes too restrictive). Hospitalization is the main form of care that HMOs intentionally tried to restrict because it is obviously so much more expensive than care provided in the doctor's office.

Curiously, even though employers had seen little evidence that managed care was reducing costs during the decade of the 1980s, they suddenly became convinced that managed care was the way to go during the 1990s. They began dropping traditional insurance as an alternative in the health care benefit package they were offering to employees. In 1993, about half of all American workers (versus the population as a whole) were enrolled in managed care programs; by 1995, that figure leaped to 73 percent.[1] The speed of the shift surprised everyone. While the pros and cons regarding the impact of managed care continued to mount, the number of people enrolled in managed care plans increased steadily throughout the 1990s. Enrollment peaked in 1999 at 30.1 percent of the population and fell to 26.4 percent by 2002.[2] You might think that this would have brought more stable, if not lower, health insurance premiums. Not so! Annual premiums continued to rise, in fact, at double-digit percentage rates during a period when the rate of inflation was around 3 percent. The average premium in 2003 was $3,383 for single coverage and $9,068 for family coverage, which explains why employers are eager to drop insurance coverage if they can while others shift more of the cost to employees.[3]

While managed care did not introduce business practices into the health care sector, the growth of managed care organizations certainly accelerated the application of such practices. Managed care organizations were interested in experimenting with a range of business management tools, most notably, software programs that monitor doctors' practice patterns. Collecting and analyzing such information permitted managed care organizations to press doctors to cut the number of patient visits, control the use of expensive tests, and generally reduce expenses associated with treatment.

Another important change brought about by the growth of managed care is the consolidation of organizations in the health sector. As managed care organizations became larger and more powerful, they were able to demand better deals in negotiations with hospitals and all the companies from which they ordered equipment and supplies (economies of scale). In many cases, managed care organizations could and ultimately did simply buy out their suppliers (vertical integration). This created even larger and more powerful organizations.

Those who favor the expansion of managed care interpreted this to mean that the most successful managed care organizations were putting the less successful ones out of business because the successful ones were clearly offering a better product. This is the American way. Business executives argue that it is self-evident that "competition is healthy!" And that explains how we moved from managed care to managed competition. Managed competition was the foundational idea on which the Clinton health reform plan was based. The concept was tainted by the failure of the plan and fell into disfavor. This does not mean that competition between managed care organizations declined; indeed, it has continued to be very much alive to this day.

Managed competition has brought us larger, more efficient managed care networks. Or has it? Critics say it brought us health care monopolies. Consider the fact that five of the biggest HMOs in the country enrolled sixty-eight million persons in 2003, which is about 92 percent of all HMO enrollees, given that total enrollment was about seventy-six million or so that year.[4] The five are United Health, with 18.7 million enrollees; Wellpoint, with 14.4 million; Aetna, with 13.0 million; Anthem, with 12.6 million; and Cigna, with 11.5 million.[5]

The five top HMOs got to where they are because of numerous mergers. In the fall of 2003, Anthem announced that it was prepared to acquire Wellpoint.

Both were originally nonprofit Blue Cross–Blue Shield plans that converted to for-profit status. The decision to merge has been reviewed by the Federal Trade Commission (FTC) and states attorneys in a number of states in which both plans operate. The FTC focused on whether the merger would create an organization so large that it would constitute restraint of trade. State's attorneys were concerned that the enrollees in their states would get less attention from the bigger and more powerful plan. The final obstacle to the merger was overcome when the insurance commissioner of California approved the $16.4 billion merger in November 2004 on the condition that Anthem will invest $265 million in California programs, including increasing insurance coverage for children, funding clinics in poor areas, and training nurses.

The question that policy makers and, more to the point, the courts have been struggling with is this: Will this vastly larger organization make the delivery of health care more efficient? Put another way—are health plan mergers helping to contain costs or does consolidation of such magnitude create monopolies with the power to set prices for the purpose of enhancing profit, with no real interest in containing costs? This question has inspired some critics to note that we have entered into the era of "unmanaged competition."

Critics and supporters alike say that the primary objective of for-profit MCOs is making money. In fact, it is their "legal, ethical, and fiduciary responsibility" to do so.[6] Most observers also agree that nonprofit HMOs have no alternative but to operate by the same rules in order to survive. Accordingly, the industry as a whole refers to the money spent on medical care as the "medical-*loss* ratio." The money spent on medical care carries a negative label because of its negative impact on the bottom line. The logic that flows from that concept is obvious—cut medical care services to increase profits.

Another major criticism of managed care concerns the compensation awarded to CEOs of managed care corporations. Critics point out that the executives are getting rich by denying care to people who are sick. A case in point is the 2003 package that went to Aetna's CEO, John Rowe.[7] He received $1,042,146 in salary, a $2.2 million bonus, new stock options that are estimated to be worth $5.6 million, a $7 million cash payment on stock options, plus other compensation of nearly $400,000. Other officers of the company received huge compensation packages as well that year. One group of investors decided to take action. The United Association of Plumbers, Pipefitters, and Sprinklerfitters proposed to shareholders and the board of directors of Aetna that Rowe's compensation package be limited to $1 million and annual bonuses be linked to performance measures. The board rejected the proposal, saying that it was too rigid. The union's move was undoubtedly spurred by the company's decision to fire 10,700 employees and lay off an additional

700 over the previous year. (Is this a story that captures the essence of the battle between the haves and have-nots or what?!)

The fact that the public continues to be dissatisfied about the rising cost of care—but has been even more dissatisfied about the restrictions imposed by HMOs aimed at controlling costs—led to the rise of PPOs (preferred provider organizations).[8] This option is presented as a flexible plan that allows employees to select less-inclusive and less-expensive options. It is consistent with the new emphasis on "consumer-driven health care." Some critics say that these plans work to help employers justify passing on a greater proportion of the premium to employees. Economists explain it as a transfer of risk from employers to employees, that is, a shift in who bears more of the risk in making decisions about the amount of protection to seek in the event of unexpected illness. Others might look at it as a matter of rearranging the deck chairs on the Titanic since there is little reason to believe that this approach will have any positive effects on the cost containment, quality, or access.

The focus on consumer preferences indicates that HMOs have decided to go back to emphasizing the maintenance of patient health, as opposed to management of physician treatment decisions. In its latest incarnation, health maintenance is being redefined as "medical management," which is best understood as the management of patient behavior and, more precisely, the management of the behavior of high-cost, chronically ill patients.[9] Economists would say that this constitutes a shift away from attempting to control the supply side (what doctors offer) to attempting to control the demand side (what patients want).

What facilitates this shift is worth considering. The fact that health plans process such a high volume of reimbursement claims means that they have more information on the patient care process than anyone except the Centers for Medicare and Medicaid Services, the government agency that oversees Medicare claims. Indeed, the managed care industry has been creating new companies to analyze those data and has been using the results to predict the progression of patients' illnesses, identify effective interventions, and find providers who are more (as well as less) effective, all in the hope of ultimately reducing expenditures.

MANAGED CARE AND PUBLIC PROGRAMS

Medicaid is the largest budget item that virtually all states need to deal with. However, states were required to obtain permission from the Health Care Financing Administration (which was renamed the Centers for Medicare and

Medicaid Services, or CMS, as you know from the last chapter) before introducing any changes aimed at controlling costs. Congress eliminated this provision in 1997 with the passage of the Balanced Budget Act, when it took steps to combine Medicaid funds with other monies into a single grant. That gave states the right to put their Medicaid populations into managed care. Why they would wish to do so is clear. States spend about 20 percent of their budgets on Medicaid.[10]

In principle, managed care can ensure greater continuity of care since there is a "primary care manager," bureaucratic language for the primary care doctor who is responsible for coordinating a patient's care. It can hold down costs by eliminating duplication of tests, reduce the risk of complications because there is greater coordination of care, eliminate much of the inappropriate (read as costly) use of emergency rooms, and so on. Furthermore, in accepting a capitation rate, the managed care organization takes over responsibility and risk involved in managing costs. This releases the state from the burden of doing so.

The initial problem was that states had very little experience with the special challenges of enrolling this population. The Medicaid population tends to be sicker, in need of more care, but lacking the resources to pay for the things that would make the plan work—for example, transportation for office visits. Medicaid enrollees are typically less educated and more easily confused by rules governing managed care. Of course, there were also instances in which potential enrollees were being intentionally misled about the rules by unscrupulous organizations hired to recruit them. Also, there was no track record to tell managed care organizations how to set the capitation rate. As a result, enrolling Medicaid populations in managed care turned out to be very problematic: patient care suffered, and everyone involved became frustrated and discouraged. After the first few years, most states learned from their mistakes, succeeded in enrolling most eligible people, and even produced better health outcomes.

Then there is the Medicare population. Remember, this is the over-sixty-five population plus some other special categories of recipients. We know that those over sixty-five are staying healthier longer, are generally not poor, and are politically active.

When the CMS analysts looked into it, they found that two very different kinds of people were enrolling in Medicare HMOs. One category included those with few health problems who joined because managed care is less costly. They had nothing to lose because, if and when they did become seriously ill, they could disenroll and go back to their private doctors for care. Needless to say, the HMOs did not mind. The second category of persons who

signed up included the chronically ill. They did so because Medicare managed care plans covered their medications. When the analysts set to find out
how much money was being saved, they found that they were overpaying for
the care of the persons in the first category and therefore cut reimbursements.[11] Managed care organizations responded by getting out of the
Medicare business in droves. They said that they could not provide the broad
coverage they had been offering to those in the second category without the
cushion of the extra funds they were receiving for enrolling all those healthy
people in the first category.

Attempts to enroll the Medicare-eligible population in the newest version
of Medicare managed care—that is, Medicare + Choice or Medicare Advantage—have been mixed.[12] Those who have not joined say that they are not interested, because they do not want to give up the right to choose their own
doctors. They would also have to give up the right to self-refer themselves to
a doctor, possibly someone who has been caring for them for years. In other
words, why should they give up something they like and have become accustomed to? Because senior citizens are so well informed about their health
care arrangements and so politically active, politicians have not tried to force
them to enroll in managed care.

As you recall from the last chapter, the 2003 drug prescription legislation
will increase the amount of money it pays HMOs to help them increase en-
rollments. According to state representative Pete Stark (D-California), the law
"lavishes billions of dollars" on HMOs. He also objected to the fact that $46
billion is to come out of the Medicare trust fund, which supports the hospital
portion of Medicare (i.e., Part A); it is a move that, as you may also recall, is
projected to bankrupt the trust fund by 2019.[13]

WHAT ABOUT THE QUALITY OF CARE?

Since an increasing number of employers have dropped traditional insurance
as an alternative to managed care, the proportion of people enrolled in HMOs
continued to grow into the late 1990s, bringing with it a rising tide of concern
regarding the impact that cost control was having on the quality of care. Policy makers worried that managed care organizations were sacrificing quality
in their efforts to reduce costs. A large number of studies have been carried in
response to this question. The results have not been conclusive but have generally not found differences significant enough to recommend action.[14]

During the mid-1990s, politicians responded to the public's concerns about
the effect of managed care organization decisions on quality by enacting leg-

islation intended to impose control over managed care organizations. This became known as the backlash era (i.e., against managed care). Nine hundred laws affecting managed care were enacted by the states between 1994 and 1998.[15] This is when the legislation we discussed in the chapter on hospitals (chapter 4) was enacted to prevent "drive through" deliveries and outpatient mastectomies. MCOs were required to allow women to stay in the hospital for two days after giving birth and to stay overnight after a mastectomy. Other laws focused on newly instituted managerial policies designed to cut costs. For example, as of 1995, states began passing laws prohibiting managed care organizations from terminating doctors "without just cause." This is in reaction to reports that doctors were fired not because they were providing poor care but because the treatments they prescribed were too expensive. By the end of 1996, eighteen states passed laws prohibiting "gag rules." This refers to restrictions on what doctors can say to patients about alternative, possibly more expensive but better forms of treatment. States also began requiring disclosure of incentives offered to doctors for cutting costs.

Fearing more direct government control, the managed care industry created its own monitoring system in the form of an accrediting organization. The National Committee for Quality Assurance (NCQA) began reviewing and accrediting HMOs and managed care organizations in 1990. During the first few years of operation, accreditation, which is voluntary, cost approximately $40,000. NCQA began by using a survey covering approximately sixty performance measures, including such things as patient satisfaction, rates of utilization of services, and organizational finances. Not exactly quality-of-care measures, but there were few universally accepted measures of quality at that time. So, NCQA created and employed a software program eventually favored by many large employers: a "report card" to gauge the performance of service providers.

The use of report cards has not come about without rancor. Doctors, hospitals, and managed care organizations all protested. For their part, many researchers interested in quality measures concluded that the report cards were of little value because they focused on a small range of indicators. Furthermore, by giving a whole practice a single score, they did not distinguish among plans because doctors generally associate themselves with several plans—so you still could not determine which doctors were better on an individual basis. Even though these early information-gathering efforts were flawed, the effort itself had interesting effects. It made information more accessible to the public. NCQA created a website that allows anyone who is interested to look up the quality report on any plan that the organization has evaluated, assuming the plan has agreed to have its evaluation released.

Government agencies, which are traditionally reluctant to release standardized data, have been doing so. It inspired other organizations to create websites of their own. The AMA, American Association of Health Plans, and the Agency for Healthcare Research and Quality sponsor websites designed to offer practice guidelines for health care professionals. Many direct patients to websites designed for them. The mushrooming of sites has been inspired in large part by the emergence of "evidence-based medicine" and the practice guidelines that flow from clinical research.

Some observers think this is all to the good because it indicates that everyone involved is now more willing to cooperate in efforts to measure quality. However, it is still not clear whether this information is being used well and, as far as patients are concerned, used at all. Employers have not paid much attention to quality measures in selecting health plans in the past. And all the evidence indicates that patients prefer to rely on personal recommendations of family, friends, and trusted doctors.

CONCLUSION

Who do you think presents a stronger case—the advocates or the critics of managed care? Clearly, your answer must lean more heavily on the theoretical perspective that reflects your worldview than on incontrovertible data. Why? Because the evidence on trends and their effects is not so clear that it is accepted without argument. There is so much data that one can pick and choose the evidence to fit a personal perspective.

For example, the managed care industry has taken full credit for stabilizing health care costs during the 1990s. There is no question that managed care worked to restrict enrollees' choices. When costs began to rise toward the end of the 1990s, the explanation offered by managed care executives was that the public was demanding more choice and less "management" over health care services, and that is precisely what drove up costs. Is it possible that managed care was only partially responsible for containing costs during the first half of the 1990s and that the improvements in technology might deserve a substantial portion of the credit?[16] Remember that laser surgery began to shorten hospital stays for many procedures around this time. Additionally, the price of computers, including those used by health care organizations, dropped more than anyone expected. The productivity of American workers in general increased, again more than anyone expected, probably due to greater reliance on computers. In fact, most sectors of the economy did better—that is, were more productive. So, does managed care deserve the credit for stabilizing costs, or did it just happen to be there at the right time to benefit?

With questions such as this in mind, let's move on to the topic of cost control and see what that evidence looks like.

NOTES

1. Gail Jensen, Michael Morrisey, Shannon Gaffney, and Derek Liston, "The New Dominance of Managed Care: Insurance Trends in the 1990s," *Health Affairs* 16 (January/February 1997): 125–36.

2. "Persons Enrolled in Health Maintenance Organizations (HMOs) by Geographic Region and State: United States, Selected Years 1980–2002," (Washington, D.C.: U.S. Department of Health and Human Services, Public Health Service, 2003), table 150.

3. Henry J. Kaiser Family Foundation, *Trends and Indicators in the Changing Health Care Market Place,* updated (Menlo Park, Calif.: 2004), exhibit 3.1.

4. "Persons Enrolled in Health Maintenance Organizations."

5. James Robinson, "From Managed Care to Consumer Health Insurance: The Fall and Rise of Aetna," *Health Affairs* 23 (March/April, 2004): 50.

6. Mark Hall and Christopher Conover, "The Impact of Blue Cross Conversions on Accessibility, Affordability, and the Public Interest," *Milbank Quarterly* 81 (2003): 509–42.

7. Robert Kazel, "Union Seeks to Limit Aetna Execs' Pay," *American Medical News* (April 12, 2004): 20.

8. Robert Hurley, Bradley Strunk, and Justin White, "The Puzzling Popularity of the PPO," *Health Affairs* 23 (March/April, 2004): 56–68.

9. James Robinson and Jill Yegin, "Medical Management after Managed Care," *Health Affairs* web exclusive (May 19, 2004): 269–80.

10. "2000–2001 State Health Care Expenditure Report," copublished by the Milbank Memorial Fund, the National Association of State Budget Officers, and the Reforming States Group (New York: April 2003), 11.

11. *Medicare HMOs: Rapid Enrollment Growth Concentrated in Selected States,* report to the Honorable John F. Kerry, U.S. Senate (Washington, D.C.: General Accounting Office, 1996).

12. *Medicare HMOs: HCFA Can Promptly Eliminate Hundreds of Millions in Excess Payments, 1997,* report to the chairman of the Subcommittee on Health, Committee on Ways and Means, House of Representatives (Washington, D.C.: General Accounting Office).

13. Markian Hawryluk, "Medicare Faces Cash Crunch," *American Medical News* (April 5, 2004): 8.

14. Bruce Landon, Alan Zaslavsy, Shulamit Bernard, Matthew Cioffi, and Paul Cleary, "Comparison of Performance of Traditional Medicare vs. Medicare Managed Care," *Journal of the American Medical Association* 291 (April 14, 2004): 1744–52.

15. Thomas Bodenheimer, "The HMO Backlash—Righteous or Reactionary?" *New England Journal of Medicine* 335 (November 21, 1996): 1601–4; Eugene Declercq

and Diana Simmes, "The Politics of 'Drive-Through Deliveries': Putting Early Post-partum Discharge on the Legislative Agenda," *Milbank Quarterly* 75 (1997): 175–202.

16. Susan Dentzer, "Honey, I Shrunk the Price Tag! Do Plunging Prices for High-Tech Help to Explain Low Inflation?" *U.S. News & World Report* 121 (September 23, 1996): 72.

9

Health Care Costs and Cost Containment

While growth in the rate of Medicare spending over the past 35 years has been impressive, if these rates of growth are projected over the next half century, the results are alarming. Over the next 75 years, for example, the proportion of the gross domestic product spent on Medicare is projected by the trustees of the Part A trust fund to grow from 2.24% to 8.6%. Other analysts claim that by 2030, Medicare will consume one-quarter of the federal budget, up from 11% in 1995.

Timothy Stoltzfus Jost
Disentitlement? The Threats Facing Our Public Health-Care Programs and a Rights-Based Response (2003)

Fiscal good times have receded; during the past three years, states have faced serious budget choices. One of the primary causes of states' financial crises from 2001 to 2004 has been the continued growth in Medicaid spending combined with falling tax revenues. Between 2001 and 2002 state Medicaid spending grew by 11.6 percent, while state tax revenues declined by 4.7 percent.

Stephen Zuckerman, Joshua McFeeter,
Peter Cunningham, and Len Nichols
Health Affairs, web exclusive
June 23, 2004

This chapter looks at how much we are spending on health care and what we are spending it on. It goes on to explore the reasons why cost containment is difficult to achieve. One explanation is, as some less-than-optimistic policy analysts have been quick to note, that you can have any two out of the three health system goals—quality, access, and cost containment—but not all three at the same time. But we as Americans insist on all three. This has left the structure of the health care system, which requires a delicate balance in the best of times, looking shaky and periodically at risk of imminent collapse.

Remember the discussion on public opinion in chapter 3, where we examined survey data on how Americans respond when asked what they think about health care costs? We found that Americans think that their personal costs are too high but that the national rate of expenditure could, and probably should, be higher. Thus far, no one has figured out how to design a policy that would achieve that objective. The difficulty is that the public does not expect increased national expenditures on health care to translate into higher taxes. Americans are convinced that more money can be found through the redistribution of current government expenditures. A closer look at the 2005 federal budget (table 9.1) submitted by the White House, but not passed at the time of this writing, makes clear why cutting other components of the budget to shift money to health care is so much more difficult than popular wisdom would suggest. The 2005 budget is very similar to the budget that was enacted in 2004 but very different from budgets enacted during periods when we were not at war.

The cost of the Iraq War has been revised a number of times, so we should expect the proportion allocated to defense to edge up some more. You should also know that several of the biggest items in the budget cannot be reduced because they are entitlements, meaning that the allocated funds must be distributed by law to categories of persons who are entitled to them. This includes social security, Medicare, and income security or pensions. The interest on debt (like interest on everyone's credit card) must also be paid to the nation's cred-

Table 9.1.   Federal Budget Proposed for 2005

Social security	21.5%
Defense	18.7
Income security entitlements (jobless benefits and pensions)	15.5
Medicare	12.3
Health	10.5
Interest on debt	7.4
Education, training, social services	3.7
Veterans benefits and services, transportation, justice, international affairs, environment, space, other	10.4
Total	*100.0*

Source: Office of the President of the United States, "Budget of the United States: Historical Tables, Fiscal Year, 2005."

itors. That leaves us with the difficult task of nominating portions that are "discretionary" for cutting, which are obviously already pretty small.

Recognizing how difficult it is to reallocate federal funds should make clear why the public's preference for increasing the proportion of the public budget dedicated to health care is so challenging. Furthermore, analysts in the Office of the Actuary (Centers for Medicare and Medicaid Services) predict that if we continue to spend on health care at the current rate, then the health share of the GDP (the federal budget is part of the total GDP) will rise from 14.9 percent in 2002 to 18.4 percent by 2013.[1] That means that cuts will have to be made in those discretionary budget categories that are already small.

Most of us look at the actual amount of money currently being spent on health care, $1,424.5 billion in 2001, and just can't comprehend it. That is undoubtedly why most of us cannot get up much enthusiasm for discussing the total amount of money involved. It is just too hard to wrap one's mind around it. The whole issue is easier to understand if we look at where the money goes in percentage terms, as outlined in table 9.2.

Given the distribution of expenditures and keeping in mind that policy makers are interested in cutting public expenditures, which categories would you expect them to cut? Policy makers have consistently gone for the biggest categories because cuts there produce the biggest impact. That makes hospital costs and physician services the main cost-cutting targets. The problem that anyone who has tried to cut hospital and physician costs quickly discovers, and as HMOs have repeatedly discovered, is that the people who complain that costs are too high are also the first to complain when they need care

Table 9.2.   U.S. Health Expenditures, Percent Distribution for 2001

Personal health care	86.8%
Hospital care	*31.7*
Professional services	*32.5*
Nursing home and home health	*9.3*
Retail sales of medical products	*13.4*
Government administration and cost of private health insurance	6.3
Government public health activities	3.3
Research and construction	3.6
Total	*100.0*

Source: "National Health Expenditures, Average Annual Percent Change, and Percent Distribution, according to Type of Expenditure: United States, Selected Years 1960–2001," *Health United States, 2003* (Washington, D.C.: U.S. Department of Health and Human Services, Public Health Service, 2003), table 115.
Note: Percentages may not add up due to rounding.

and cannot get it. Cutting back on the cost of hospitalization and physician services quickly translates into cuts in services to patients, which is definitely not well received by the public.

To be more specific, what we discovered in chapter 3 is that Americans are primarily concerned about their out-of-pocket costs. The out-of-pocket distribution looks somewhat different from the distribution in table 9.2. The largest share of the 2002 health care dollar coming out of our pockets goes to prescription drugs at 22.9 percent; next comes physician services at 16.1 percent; and dental care at 14.5 percent. The share of consumer personal income going to cover out-of-pocket health care costs is projected to increase from 2.7 percent in 2002 to 3.1 percent by 2013. This appears to be a small difference, but the historical record indicates that it matters. When out-of-pocket costs hit 3.2 percent in 1974 and in 1990, the public demanded that the government act to do something about health care costs. HMO legislation was enacted in 1974, and health care reform topped the political agenda leading to the 1992 presidential election.[2]

COST CONTAINMENT OPTIONS

Writing at the height of the Clinton administration reform debates, Victor Fuchs, a highly respected economist, captured the essence of the difficulty in identifying effective cost containment measures. He borrowed a maxim made famous by Jane Fonda, who was promoting her exercise video at around that time: "No pain, no gain." Fuchs said that we have only three options if we wish to reduce costs: institute cuts in the prices we pay for health services; reduce services to patients; and produce and deliver health services at a lower cost.[3] As you know, most people would like to see the cost of health care decrease; it is just that we cannot agree on how to achieve that.

According to Fuchs, the first option is the least promising. He pointed out that savings achieved by cutting the prices to pharmaceutical companies (which have extremely high profits) or doctors' incomes (which are higher than those of their colleagues in many other countries) would be small. He calculated that reducing drug company profits by 50 percent would decrease health care expenditures by less than 1 percent.

Fuchs went on to say that a version of the second option provided the ideal solution—that is, cutting patient services that are not efficacious. However, this requires distinguishing the treatments that are effective from those that are ineffective. Agencies of the federal government plus private foundations have been funding "outcome" research and have been outlining "evidence-based" practice patterns designed to identify the treatments that produce the most successful results. The reasoning here is that the quality of care will be preserved while the search for cost-cutting targets continues. However, this strategy is not easy to implement, according to Fuchs, because "low yield" medicine is not "no yield" medicine. Some less-than-productive treatments are not eliminated, because patients insist on them even though such treatments do not produce much objective benefit.

At this point, the third option, producing services at a lower cost may look like a sure winner, but it turns out to inspire the most controversy. Here we get into matters connected to "production costs." Cutting personnel costs via "downsizing" and "reengineering" have become familiar tactics used by major corporations. As you know, based on chapter 4, health care delivery organizations used the same approach with mixed results and reactions from a range of observers. We know that for the past few decades nurses bore the brunt of layoffs and were replaced with employees who were considerably less expensive because they came to this work with considerably less education and training. This solution has not worked, because hospitals have been admitting sicker patients than before whose care is more complicated and requires staff with more advanced skills.

Another way to reduce production costs is to keep the clinical staff but get rid of the office staff who do not have direct patient care responsibilities. This solution targets administrative costs. According to two doctors based at Harvard University Medical School, Steffie Woolhandler and David Himmelstein, who have been analyzing health care delivery issues for some time, the United States spends about twenty-five cents out of every health care dollar on administrative expenses.[4] How is that possible? According to the two analysts, the money is largely wasted on clerical staff who fill out insurance forms—in the insurance company office, the doctor's office, and the hospital billing department. The work of processing insurance claims begins with calls to the insurance company to check whether the procedure is covered; then there is the follow-up paperwork, including billing the patient separately for service provided that carries a co-payment. Since coverage is continually revised, mistakes are common and create more phone calls because each insurance company—and there were still about 1,250 of them operating in the United States at the end of the 1990s—had its own plan, often multiple plans, each with its own restrictions. Furthermore, there were four hundred kinds of formats for submitting insurance information.[5] Each claim presents a new challenge. The number of plans and forms may have decreased, but that has not had much impact on administrative costs.

The solution according to Woolhandler and Himmelstein, among others, is to do what virtually all the other highly advanced industrialized countries have done: reduce administrative costs by consolidating and simplifying arrangements, which would be achieved by establishing a national health plan. This would, of course, involve the federal government. However, many Americans think that relying on the government is likely to result in greater inefficiency and higher costs. The logic behind this firmly held belief would lead one to expect that all those other countries pay more for health care services because their governments have played a greater role in their respective systems. However, we know that is not true. Not only do Americans believe that the government is inefficient, but Americans are also certain that a government-sponsored health plan would mean higher taxes—and we strongly believe that we pay too much in taxes already. The question this raises is, How much are we being taxed compared to people in other countries?

ARE WE TAXING OURSELVES TOO MUCH OR TOO LITTLE?

In 1998, our taxes were lower than those in twenty-five of the most economically advanced countries in the world that are members of the Organization for Economic Cooperation and Development (the OECD tracks development in thirty of the most highly industrialized countries in the world).[6] In 2001, the percent of the GDP coming from taxes was 25 percent in the United States; by contrast, it was 45 percent in France, 37 percent in the United Kingdom, 37 percent in Germany, and 35 percent in Canada; only Japan, out of the seven most advanced nations, had a lower tax rate, at 24 percent.[7] In short, our taxes are clearly lower than are taxes in most countries. It is worth noting, however, that our taxes buy us a lot less government-supported health care than government spending achieves in nearly all other countries. The U.S. government covers only 45 percent of health care costs while governments in other countries cover about 74 percent.

What explains why we pay more for health care services in this country but receive less for our health care dollars is easy to explain according to some analysts. The basic reason, they say, is that we pay higher prices for those services than do people in other countries.[8] How we might alter that situation is the problem. This is where the debate turns back to the question of who is better equipped to control costs—the government or the private sector. We will address this topic in some detail in chapter 11, where we turn to debates on health care reform.

CONCLUSION

Whenever the problems confronting the health care system move to the center of public debate, it seems that Americans can agree that costs are too high, but they find little to agree on after that. The reason is that this social institution, like all the others, must operate as a reflection of our values and beliefs about the best approach for responding to society's wants and needs regarding health care services. Americans apply those values in considering the basic questions raised by discussions on health care cost containment. We differ in our attitudes regarding who should ultimately be responsible for reducing costs, how we should pay for what it does cost, who should qualify for the benefits, should the benefits be the same for everyone, and so forth.

It is worth noting that reasonable representatives of alternative positions in these debates have begun to admit that their respective approaches are not perfect. In the end, all of us must decide which set of imperfections we would prefer to live with. This is complicated by the fact that accurate information is not always easy to obtain. Too often, the information being presented is incomplete. More disturbing is the extent to which totally distorted information is reported and passed on by those whose ideological commitment is so strong that they are willing to dismiss inconvenient facts that get in the way. There is no question about it: the "reality" that people on all sides of these debates cite in presenting their solutions for containing health care costs is "constructed."

As I have said, arguments about accurately interpreting the relevant facts is what makes health care reform so much of an uphill battle. Before we consider the solutions to the problems that confront the U.S. health care delivery system and the solutions being proposed to deal with those problems—that is, health care reform—it might be interesting to consider the health care arrangements that exist in other countries. That is the focus of the following chapter.

NOTES

1. Stephen Heffler, Sheila Smith, Sean Keehan, M. Kent Clemens, Mark Zezza, and Christopher Truffer, "Health Spending Projections Through 2013," *Health Affairs* web exclusive (February 11, 2004): 79–93.

2. "Gross Domestic Product, Federal and State and Local Government Expenditures, National Health Expenditures, and Average Annual Percent Change: United States, Selected Years 1960–2001," *Health United States, 2003* (Washington, D.C.: U.S. Department of Health and Human Services, Public Health Service, 2003), table 112. "National Health Expenditures, Average Annual Percent Change, and Percent Distribution, according to Type of Expenditure: United States, Selected Years 1960–2001," *Health United States, 2003* (Washington, D.C.: U.S. Department of Health and Human Services, Public Health Service, 2003), table 115.

3. Victor Fuchs, "No Pain, No Gain," *Journal of the American Medical Association* 269 (February 3, 1993): 631–33.

4. Steffie Woolhandler and David Himmelstein, "Costs of Care and Administration at For-Profit and Other Hospitals in the United States," *New England Journal of Medicine* 336 (March 13, 1997): 769–74.

5. John Iglehart, "Health Policy Report: Private Insurance," *New England Journal of Medicine* 326 (June 18, 1992): 1715–20.

6. Organization for Economic Cooperation and Development, *Tax and the Economy: A Comparative Assessment of OECD Countries,* Tax Policy Studies 6 (Paris: Organization for Economic Cooperation and Development, 2001).

7. Organization for Economic Cooperation and Development, *Revenue Statistics, 1965–2002* unpublished data (Paris: Organization for Economic Cooperation and Development).

8. Heffler and others, "Health Spending Projections"; Gerard Anderson, Uwe Reinhardt, Peter Hussey, and Varduhi Petrosyan, "It's the Prices, Stupid: Why the United States Is So Different from Other Countries," *Health Affairs* 22 (May/June): 89–105.

10

The Health Care Systems in Other Countries

In 2000 the United States spent considerably more on health care than any other country, whether measured per capital or as a percentage of GDP. At the same time, most measures of aggregate utilization such as physician visits per capita and hospital days per capita were below the OECD [Organization for Economic Cooperation and Development] median. Since spending is a product of both the goods and services used and their prices, this implies that much higher prices are paid in the United States than in other countries. But U.S. policymakers need to reflect on what Americans are getting for their greater health spending. They could conclude: It's the prices, stupid.

Gerard F. Anderson, Uwe E. Reinhardt,
Peter Hussey, and Varduhi Petroysan
Health Affairs
May/June, 2003

The most recent Commonwealth Fund International Health Policy Survey asked hospital executives in five countries — Australia, Canada, New Zealand, the United Kingdom, and the United States — for their views of their nation's health care system. . . .

The survey found a higher rate of dissatisfaction among U.S. hospital executives even though they were more likely than their counterparts to report a strong financial situation, excellent facilities, resources available to expand or improve current services, and short waiting times, or none at all, for elective surgery.

U.S. hospital executives also stood out as being the most concerned about market competition, the expense of providing care to the uninsured, and the cost of malpractice insurance. Furthermore, U.S. hospital executives were the most reluctant to disclose quality-of-care data to the public.

Commonwealth Fund
Publication no. 747
May 2004

Scholars in virtually all highly industrialized countries have been studying health care arrangements in other countries for good reason. All countries are experiencing steadily rising costs and are struggling to identify mechanisms that will reduce costs without a negative effect on quality. The more specific question that American scholars struggle with is why we are not achieving better health outcomes given how much we spend. While data on comparative expenditures are far easier to come by than data on satisfaction and quality, there is still an overwhelming amount of information to sift through. To make this task more manageable, we will examine data on four countries—the United Kingdom, Canada, Germany, and Japan. Why those four? Because people in this country have at various times used the first three to illustrate how making changes would make our health care system either far better or far worse. I include Japan because, since the early 1980s, it has had the lowest infant mortality rate and highest life expectancy rate of any country in the world. (Hong Kong, which has only recently been included in such comparisons, has been in first or second place over the last few years.) Not that anyone in this country has suggested adopting the Japanese system, however, it is still worth considering what accounts for their good health—and, more specifically, to consider the extent to which their health system can be credited for it.

To open the discussion, table 10.1 shows the basic measures of health and national expenditures for each of these four countries as the major descriptive characteristics against which we will be comparing the countries' health care delivery systems.

Table 10.1. Life Expectancy, Infant Mortality, and Expenditures per Gross Domestic Product (GDP)

	Life expectancy[a]		Infant mortality[a]	GDP	U.S. GDP[b]
Japan	77.2M	84.0F	3.4	8.0%	44%
UK	75.1	80.0	5.8	7.6	41
Canada	76.0	81.5	5.3	9.7	57
Germany	74.5	80.6	4.5	10.7	57
U.S.	73.8	79.5	7.1	13.9	100

[a]*Health United States, 2003* (Washington, D.C.: U.S. Department of Health and Human Services), tables 25 and 26. Figures are for the years 1998 (life expectancy) and 1999 (infant mortality).
[b]Uwe Reinhardt, Peter Hussey, and Gerard Anderson, "U.S. Health Care Spending in an International Context," *Health Affairs* 23 (May/June, 2004): 10–25. Both GDP columns are for the year 2001.

THE UNITED KINGDOM

The United Kingdom includes England, Scotland, Wales, and Northern Ireland. Because the health care systems are not identical throughout the United Kingdom, the following discussion focuses on England, where health insurance for workers came into existence about 1911. Health care for the worker's family was the family's responsibility. The logic here is clear. Remember, England was where the industrial revolution began. The industrialists were interested in making sure that their workers had access to health care services. Their main concern was workforce stability, not anyone's health per se and certainly not the health of persons who were not their employees.

The emergence of hospitals in England has a long history that serves as a particularly graphic illustration of how social values influence the development of social institutions.[1] Hospitals were established several centuries ago (some as early as the sixteenth and seventeenth centuries) with the express purpose of serving three segments of the population. The aristocracy went to sanatoriums, which were located in the countryside where the patients could benefit from clean air and the special comforts expected by the rich. The working poor (i.e., all workers, in contrast to the aristocracy who do not work even now) went to voluntary hospitals, often operated by religious orders. That left the "undeserving poor" (i.e., those who were too sick, too old, too disabled to work). Because the aristocracy would not mix with the working poor nor with the undeserving poor, each segment had to have its own hospital. All that changed with World War II.

During the war, the government mapped out all the hospitals and counted all the hospital beds in the country and mandated that 10 percent of the beds in each hospital be set aside for military use. The hospitals were paid a per diem rate whether the bed was in use or not. Everyone in the country was making sacrifices. This was the hospitals' contribution to the war effort. While the country came out of the war victorious, it sustained heavy damage and was broke. The government proposed taking over responsibility for the entire health care system as a reward to the public for making enormous sacrifices during the wartime period. In other words, from that time on, the government took over ownership of the whole health care system. Not everyone was entirely happy about this plan. Doctors were especially loud in their objections. They said the government's plan was socialized medicine and would bring with it the downfall of professional medical practice. Objectively, it was, for better or worse, a major step toward socialized medicine. Doctors objected to being salaried instead of being paid as professionals under the traditional fee-for-service arrangement. However, one has to be practical in these matters. Having the government provide a guaranteed income was not easy to dismiss given the postwar state of affairs.

The solution was interesting. The general practitioners agreed to being paid under a capitation arrangement. They agreed to having X number of patients, usually around two thousand, more or less depending on whether the practice was in an urban or rural area; the patients would sign up with them for care, and the doctors would get paid "by the head" (i.e., via capitation) whether those patients came to see them or not. This meant that the doctors were guaranteed a steady income. The patients were guaranteed the services of a doctor. Patients had the opportunity to change doctors once a year by signing up with a new doctor of their choice. The specialists made a different bargain. They agreed to be salaried and work for a particular hospital in return for having access to 10 percent of the beds in that hospital for their private patients, whom they could bill separately. Everyone else working in the hospital had always been salaried, so that did not change.

In short, as of 1948, England has had a National Health Service (NHS), not a national health insurance system. Everyone in the country has had full access to health care services since then. In assuming responsibility for the hospitals as of 1948, the government took over ownership of all the hospitals and clinics. It pays everyone who works for the NHS. How happy is everyone involved? How can you tell? When asked, the British have said that the health care system is second only to the monarchy in popularity.[2] This should not be taken to mean that they do not complain about the system. A more concrete way of assessing satisfaction is to count how many people opt out of the system. In the case of doctors, how many choose to leave to practice elsewhere? The critics of the NHS say that doctors are leaving in droves. In actuality, it is difficult to know how many leave and for what reasons. There is no concrete evidence to indicate that any significant number leave. There is also no count of how many leave and return after some period of postgraduate education or research outside the country (not always to the United States). To the extent that evidence exists, very few doctors are leaving.

In the case of patients, the measure is how many choose to buy private insurance and go to private doctors and hospitals. Until the 1980s, only about 5 percent of the population chose to buy private insurance. By the early 1990s, about 15 percent had done so. That figure has not changed much since then. How should we interpret this? It certainly indicates some growth in dissatisfaction but not wholesale growth, right? There is another catch here that is worth noting.

When people buy private insurance, they buy it on top of having access to care through the NHS. What advantage are people seeking in buying private insurance if they have access to free care? Better doctors, better technology, more care? Not exactly. The answer is that they are getting around the "queue." To keep costs down, the NHS prevents people from getting health care services "on demand" (i.e., whenever they feel like it) for problems that are not life threatening. In other words, people must wait while more urgent cases are treated. Those who believe that the wait is too long, and can afford to do so, buy private insurance. One of the most often-cited reasons for doing this has been hip replacement surgery. This condition is painful but not life threatening.

Now for the essence of the "catch" I mentioned earlier. Private hospitals, where patients with private insurance go, do routine surgeries, such as hip replacements. (I know, not "routine" to the person having the surgery but routine in terms of how often it is done and how much risk is involved.) If something does go seriously wrong, the patient is picked up by ambulance and taken to a major NHS hospital, which is equipped to deal with high-risk and complicated problems. So everyone is happy right? Well, not entirely.

The reason that people have been buying private insurance is that the government had kept the budget for the NHS low—much too low in the opinion of some. (England spent about half of what we spent for the last two decades of the twentieth century as reflected in percentage of GDP.) Couldn't the British alter this; after all, it is their social institution—they created it, they can change it, right? That is true. But remember this is the NHS, not an insurance plan. Its budget is in the hands of the ruling political party in office, which is elected by the public. In theory, the public should be able to persuade the government to respond to its demands and allocate more funds for this purpose. The public did demand increased funding during the 1980s, and on one or two occasions the government did respond but only after an enormous amount of public protest. The NHS did not receive a major infusion of funds until 1998, after the British chose to elect a new prime minister in 1997, Tony Blair, who promised to put more liberal policies in place, including allocating more funding for the health care system. Since people must weigh their dissatisfaction with the way one social institution is being treated by the government against how they think other social institutions are faring, they may not be so eager to oust the current party until they are sufficiently unhappy about all of it. They are more apt to try to persuade the government via appeals and protests first. In 1997, British citizens did determine that electing a more liberal political party to office would improve the health care system as well as other social arrangements and institutions.

Blair has been true to his word.[3] His objective was to raise the NHS budget from the 6.8 percent of GDP spent in 1997 to 9.4 percent by 2007–2008. Blair made clear that he would reverse the changes introduced during the two previous Conservative Party administrations, lead by Margaret Thatcher and

John Major, who had been impressed with U.S. efforts to introduce competition to increase efficiency. The mechanism the Conservative administrations had designed to promote greater efficiency was "fund holding." This gave general practitioners the option of managing their own funds and spending the monies they saved in running the practice on anything the practice group wanted to purchase. (They could not keep the surplus as a bonus.) Policy makers were somewhat surprised to find that the groups used the funds to ensure that social services were more closely aligned with medical services. The American way would have been to spend it on more technology and more expensive furnishings for their offices to attract more patients. Right? The British apparently hold public good in higher regard than private gain, which just goes to show how cultural values shape social institutions and why they vary from one country to another.

Tony Blair set out to abolish fund holding, with the aim of promoting cooperation rather than competition. The change turned out to be semantic. What changed was what physician practice groups are called—from fund holders to primary care trusts. Additionally, participation became compulsory. A number of other, more sweeping changes followed, including availability of funds for additional personnel plus funds for the construction of new medical schools. New diagnostic and treatment centers were opened to reduce waiting times. A National Institute for Clinical Excellence was established and mandated to issue binding recommendations on the delivery of medical services funded by the NHS. Doctors are now also required to go through relicensure every five years. The latter two changes occurred in reaction to the death of a number of children, the result of cardiac surgeons doing operations outside of their competence, which outraged the British public. The performance of each primary care trust is now rated on a star basis—zero to three—and rewarded with increased autonomy or punished through increased managerial oversight, depending on the number of stars earned. The intent is to encourage peer review and adherence to evidence-based clinical guidelines. Three-star trusts, designated "foundation trusts," are given far greater independence, allowing them to raise capital on their own rather than be totally dependent on the national treasury. All trusts are expected to move in this direction eventually.

As of April 2004, general practitioners may for the first time choose from a number of contractual incentive arrangements, including capitation with incentives for reaching particular service targets (e.g., a higher vaccination rate). This is part of an effort to reach ten specific targets for quality improvement, such as reducing cancer death by 20 percent. Contracts with specialists, called "consultants" in England, will change only to the extent that NHS patients will now schedule their own appointments with specialists online, which is likely to increase workload.

In spite of all the changes introduced and money invested into the NHS by the Blair government, 69 percent of the British public maintains that ~~gov~~ernment is not improving things enough, and physicians report that ~~they are~~ suffering from low morale.[4] British policy analysts have concluded ~~it is~~ almost as difficult to spend more money effectively in England as it is to control costs in the United States. The basic problem seems to be that expectations have been raised higher than those the government can meet.

Critics of the U.S. health care system remind us that in spite of these problems England has an enviable record of providing access to health care for everyone in the country for a very long time with a life expectancy that is higher than ours. But they can say that about most European countries without making special mention of England. There is obviously much more to say about the NHS, which does not come up for criticism in this country by those who oppose the creation of a national health care system nearly as often as it did some decades ago. When Americans argue on this point, they are far more likely to compare our health care arrangements to what they recognize as the flawed system of socialized medicine in Canada. As we all know, that position is meant to invoke images of failure, grinding bureaucracy, and incompetence. In truth, whether socialized medicine is terrible is really not the point, because Canadians do not have socialized medicine. Let's take a look at the main features of their system more closely.

CANADA

Canada has ten provinces (like American states but more independent of the federal government) and three territories (the Yukon Territory, the Northwest Territories, and Nunavut). The foundation for the eventual development of the Canadian health care system was laid in 1867, when the federal government gave the provinces responsibility for health care. However, the Canadian system really took shape during the 1940s. In 1947, the province of Saskatchewan was the first to enact a provincial hospital insurance plan. In 1957, the federal government passed legislation establishing a national program to which the provinces would have to sign on and agreed to pay for half the costs. By 1961, all the provinces had adopted the plan. The financial windfall of federal support caused Saskatchewan to propose a new program to cover medical care costs (i.e., doctors' fees). The doctors did not like the hospital plan and were vehemently opposed to the medical portion of the plan. They said that this was the beginning of socialized medicine, which would cause quality to decline, costs to go up because of mismanagement, and treatments to be determined by bureaucrats. The citizens of the province thought otherwise. Saskatchewan introduced medical insurance in 1961. The other provinces followed, and by 1971 Canada had a national health insurance program it called Medicare.

The Canadian Medicare plan has a few distinguishing features. It is generally referred to as a "single-payer" plan. The single payer is, of course, the government. Coverage must be comprehensive as specified by federal law, but additional services—such as dental benefits, home care, and drugs—are offered at the discretion of the province. The majority of hospitals are privately owned and operated by nonprofit organizations. Most doctors are paid on a fee-for-service basis, although an increasing number are opting to be paid on a salary basis. Patients are free to choose any doctor they want. They are issued a Medicare card, which is like a credit card, but see no bills because the doctors' charges are reimbursed directly by the government.

We have a lot in common with Canadians. We share a lengthy border. We speak the same language. We have similar historical roots. People in other countries cannot really tell us apart from the Canadians. So if we are so much like them and their health care arrangements seem to be superior to ours— that is, they spend less than we do, everyone is fully covered, they live a little longer than we do, and they seem to be quite satisfied—why don't we just copy it and be done with it? The answer is that no matter how alike we seem to be on the outside, the Canadian plan reflects their values, which are not our values; even if some people in this country would like for the United States to embrace their values, that is not the way it works. Consider some of the objections heard in this country.

In the Canadian system, everyone is covered by the same plan, which means you cannot buy more, faster, or better care. Americans reject that kind of arrangement. It is true that some Canadians have argued against it as well, but the majority of Canadians like things just the way they are. The position of the majority is that, when everyone is in the same boat, that boat is likely to be much better cared for. In other words, it is always easier to deny funding to "them," but when it is "us" whose care is at stake, "we" tend to exhibit more concern and readiness to treat the topic of increased funding more seriously. In Canada, you can buy more of or upgrade anything the government does not cover—better wheelchairs, eyeglasses, even more amenities in your hospital room. Selling private health insurance for anything the government covers was made illegal with the passage of Medicare. You cannot buy more technology unless you want to go across the border to the United States and pay for it out of your own pocket. The critics say that Canadians do that a lot. But what is "a lot"? And, who is doing it? Let us look at the details.

According to the Canadians, it is inefficient to buy too much technology, such as the big-ticket items like CT scanners. (Remember the discussion on the reasons behind the rising costs of hospital care in chapter 4? Technology was a big part of it.) They are very firm in sticking to a policy based on the conviction that it is better to make sure the technology you already own is fully utilized. That makes the operators more experienced and the tools more effective. When the waiting time gets too long, as it does on some occasions, Canadians must decide whether to increase funding or do without the tests, treatments, or whatever. Because so many people have a direct interest, the debates tend to be very public and very lively. In the meantime, if a particular hospital's budget allows for it, the hospital can simply contract some procedures to other hospitals that are not being fully utilized—across the border, for example. That practice is done regularly in places where U.S. hospitals are literally across town—for example, Vancouver and Seattle, or Windsor (Ontario) and Detroit. Because American hospitals have technology that is underused, they are happy to offer a reasonable rate to the Canadian hospitals on a contractual basis. So, yes, Canadians go across the border for care, but their health plan covers it, at least in some cases.

Another significant feature of the Canadian system is the cap on funding. Each year the provincial government sets a health care budget. Hospitals receive a fixed amount of money that covers basic operating expenses plus inflation, but they must negotiate any major expenses separately.

Doctors' fees are reimbursed in full for all the charges they submit. Why doesn't this result in unlimited charges? One reason is that doctors, particularly specialists, have increasingly been opting to be reimbursed on a non-fee-for-service basis. They sign a fixed annual contract with the hospital where they do most of their work. Those who rely on fee-for-service reimbursement accept lower levels of reimbursement after reaching specified income levels in some but not all provinces. As of 2004, doctors in Ontario, which is the richest province, agreed to accept 75 percent of the scheduled fee after they reach $465,000. Doctors' fee schedules are determined through negotiation between each provincial government and provincial medical society. In short, the provincial government can prepare its budget based on the record of expenditures over the previous year.

American doctors have traditionally considered Canadian reimbursement arrangements to be an unacceptable intrusion on the part of the government. Canadian doctors see it as preferable to the constant "micromanagement" that American doctors have to tolerate from managed care organizations and insurance companies. American doctors have to get preapproval from patients' insurance companies for many procedures to be sure that the insurance plan covers the procedure and that they will be paid for performing it. Because there are so many plans with so many variations in coverage that may change at any time, doctors' organizations in this country have periodically issued statements indicating support for the single-payer approach.

Another reason that explains why Canadian doctors are willing to accept a cap on income or a set salary has to do with two notable differences in expenses doctors face in the United States and Canada. U.S. doctors are more likely to enter into practice with a large educational debt. Canadian medical schools are heavily subsidized by the government, meaning that medical school tuition runs anywhere from $3,000 to $15,000 per year, depending on the province, compared to $60,000 to $125,000 per year in the United States. Also, malpractice insurance has been much lower, in part, because contingency fees are considered unethical or illegal in Canada. (A contingency fee is what lawyers charge. It is a third or quarter of the settlement, depending on whether the case is settled in or out of court, and no fee if they lose the case. U.S. lawyers argue that people could not afford to sue if lawyers charged for their time regardless of outcome.)

Because Canadians spend a lot of time criticizing the system and debating exactly what it is they want to do to make it better, the health care system is continually undergoing adjustment. That was true even while they were registering greater satisfaction with their arrangements than were people in most other countries during the early 1990s. The drop in fiscal support from the federal government, however, is what has spurred the continuing debate over the last two decades. The federal contribution to health care costs, which was originally 50 percent, was initially cut during the 1980s, finally dropping down to 25 percent by the early 1990s. With each cut, the provinces were forced to find funds to make up for the loss of federal funds. As you might imagine, talking about how to compensate for lost funds opened public debate regarding where the money should come from. This led to highly charged questions about what should be cut to lower costs and whether to allow more health care services to be offered for an additional charge. The fact that Canada was faced with an economic recession during the early 1990s led to the fear that the health care system was threatened. The economy improved during the last years of the twentieth century. In 1999, the federal government announced a fiscal surplus, which everyone agreed should go to the provinces to cover Medicare.[5]

Accordingly, as concern about funding declined, so has the volume of debate about how to best save the health care system. Polls have long found Canadians expressing strong support for maintaining the status quo on the essence of the single-payer arrangement, meaning they overwhelmingly reject two-tier care and user fees for core services. The most recent polls indicate a slight shift in readiness, especially among younger Canadians, to consider user fees for the most rapidly expanding sectors, especially newer forms of technology and home care.[6]

To sum up, the most important differences between the Canadian system and ours is that theirs is a single-payer, capped system, while ours depends on market forces and competition to control costs; theirs provides health care coverage for everyone, ours does not; and theirs costs less than ours. These points speak to costs and access, but what about quality? Their life expectancy and infant mortality rates are better than ours. This is, of course, just scratching the surface of things that people can argue about in discussing the differences between their system and our system. At this point we will consider Germany's health care system, which has been attracting more attention in recent years. It is worth remembering that German unification in 1990 produced a great deal of disruption and required a considerable investment of funds by West Germany to upgrade the East German system. The Germans say that this process has taken longer than expected and has cost more than expected.

GERMANY

The German health care system is the oldest national health care system in Europe. It was introduced in 1871 by the government under Otto Von Bismarck (in one part of Germany, Prussia), who reasoned that if the government was thought to be meeting the needs of workers as the country went through industrialization, workers would be less likely to support radical political movements and his government would stay in control. The current system took shape in 1883 with the passage of the Sickness Insurance Act and applied to all of Germany. The law required all workers below a certain income level to join existing mutual-benefit societies that had established branches that dealt with health care, called sickness funds. The law also required employees and employers to contribute to the insurance premium.

Mutual-benefit societies were created by guilds and, in some cases, villages over the last two or three hundred years to cover the costs of such catastrophes as funerals, lost income resulting from a temporary injury, and permanent disability. People set up these funds to meet the needs they thought were most pressing at the time. Coverage for health care was a secondary consideration until much later because the effectiveness of health care was limited and what was available was not costly. By the time that the Sickness Insurance Act was passed, 18,942 sickness funds were already in existence covering 4.7 million people.[7]

The 1883 law gave the funds the authority to establish and operate health clinics. This meant that they were in a position to hire doctors and other staff members. Because the sickness funds were small and were being run by persons who did not necessarily have the skill to manage large sums of money, doctors were often not paid as promised and would respond by going out on strike. The system cannot be described as stable and working to the satisfaction of all involved.[8] Things became more stable, however, during the 1930s. Interestingly, while doctors were dissatisfied with prevailing arrangements, they had little influence in shaping the national health insurance system before this time because they had no professional association to represent their views. Thus, Germany's doctors organized themselves into a national association in 1931. (Remember, the American Medical Association came into existence in 1847.)

The German health care system evolved as the society modernized, which affected the organization of the sickness funds as well. The number of funds declined over time as some failed and others merged. The number of people covered by sickness funds increased because the government lowered the minimum income level at which workers were required to enroll and employers were required to contribute. In fact, the majority of Germans joined even if they were not required to do so. By the late 1980s, over 90 percent of the population had joined. Others who earn more than the minimum income set by the government for mandatory enrollment in a sickness fund (around $40,000 by the late 1990s) may choose to buy private insurance coverage. The result is that everyone in Germany has health insurance.

Clearly the federal government has been closely involved in shaping the health care system from the beginning. As health care costs began to rise, the government introduced mechanisms designed to control costs. It separated the responsibility for day-to-day operating expenses from capital costs (new buildings, new equipment) by agreeing to cover capital expenses from government funds. It determined that operating expenses would be paid on a per diem basis, which is determined on an annual basis in negotiations that involve hospitals, sickness funds, and the government. Since 1986, hospitals have been required to operate within a preset budget that they agree to at the beginning of each year. Before then, they were paid whatever they charged. This change has had a significant stabilizing effect on rising health care costs.

Doctors are either office or hospital based. Their practices do not overlap. The hospital-based doctors are salaried. The salary is set according to the doctor's specialty and years of experience. Those rates are determined in negotiations between the sickness funds and local physicians' associations. The office-based doctors are paid on a fee-for-service basis, according to a fee schedule established in negotiations between sickness fund managers and physicians' groups. The fees are also subject to a cap, which works in response to an interesting and effective mechanism. Medical expenditures are reviewed on a quarterly basis by a unit created by the local medical society. If the total expenditures on office-based physicians' fees exceed projected funds, the fees for all office-based practitioners are reduced. Doctors whose fees are significantly higher than those of their colleagues are likely to come under scrutiny—not by bureaucrats but by a committee of fellow physicians who have the expertise as well as the authority to evaluate the reasons behind the high rate. That tends to keep the lid on fees.

It is worth noting that the German system underwent considerable change during the 1990s. Like the United Kingdom and a number of other European countries, the Germans were intrigued by the managed care experiment they saw being developed in the United States. In part, this was a response to the sudden rise in health care costs that resulted from the additional funds being expended in restructuring the system of care found in East Germany to match the highly technologically advanced system in West Germany. In 1993 and again in 1997, Germany passed legislation to promote competition among sickness funds. The legislation allowed workers greater choice of plans and instituted mechanisms to compensate for the higher costs incurred in caring for higher-risk patients. This was done to ensure that chronically ill patients were not only recruited by sickness funds (because they came with additional compensation) but were receiving treatment. Germany also instituted the Disease Management Program in 2002, which requires sickness funds to meet Ministry of Health standards of care and document treatments.

The most notable effect of the legislation promoting competition has been the rapid decrease in the number of sickness funds. Between 1993 and 2003, the number of funds dropped from 1,221 to 319.[9] Another change that took place around this time was the drop in the number of days Germans stayed in the hospital—from 15.3 days in 1990 to 11.4 days in 1997.[10] The latter is largely due to the increase in the number of procedures being carried out on an outpatient basis, which is explained by a number of factors in addition to competition. It has mostly to do with how ambulatory and hospital-based doctors divide up patient care responsibilities.

One other thing that has caused a fair amount of dissatisfaction and upset during the period the government was attempting to control costs was the reduction in access to spa treatments. The Germans are great believers in the value of the baths and massages that spas provide. In an effort to cut costs, the government urged sickness funds to reduce coverage from two weeks to ten days or even less.

In the end, Germany is willing to experiment with competition as long as it does not damage the strengths of the existing system and upset any of the major stakeholders. Put that way, one can understand why the German health care system is not changing very radically or very fast.

The German system has not been the object of nearly as much attack as the systems operating in the United Kingdom or Canada, probably because it has not been promoted by U.S. policy makers enough to threaten participants in our system who have a vested interest in keeping the system the way it is. It is also not likely to come under nearly as much attack as the Canadian system, because while it does put some restrictions on doctors' income and hospital expansion plans, it permits the coexistence of multiple insurance plans (i.e., the sickness funds). Those who are promoting it as having features the United States might adopt stress that it permits people to choose among insurance plans; that is, it does not depend on a "single payer" model, as does Canada. It allows those who can afford it to buy more insurance. It uses a negotiated cap on spending but permits a certain degree of competition under that cap. Health policy analysts say that Americans would probably be able to live with that.

JAPAN

The Japanese instituted health insurance in 1927. The country had universal coverage by 1961. The Japanese health system relies on over five thousand insurance plans to organize payment for health care services. About a quarter of the population is covered by self-funded, employer-based plans, meaning that employees and employers contribute. The proportions paid by employers and employees are similar but not identical from one employer to another. The plans are closely regulated by the government. Another 30 percent of the population is covered under employer-based plans that are government managed and partially government subsidized. The remainder of the population, which includes the self-employed and pensioners, is covered by a plan operated and subsidized by local governments. It sets premiums on the basis of family income.[11]

Americans find Japanese health care arrangements very different from ours. The differences reflect the fact that Japan built its health care system by grafting Western medical practices onto a system based on the delivery of oriental, basically Chinese, medicine. Many doctors advocate the use of herbal medications as well as pharmaceuticals used in Western medicine. They not only prescribe but dispense both kinds of medications. To put this into context, oriental medicine favors medications and discourages surgery. So there is a lot of prescribing.

The government's role in this matter is interesting. How much doctors may dispense at any one time is restricted by law. That provision suits the doctors in private practice because the patients must make return visits to obtain more drugs, but it also produces some other interesting anomalies. The clinic doctors—who own and operate private clinics, practice general medicine, and accept fees for their services—earn a great deal more than do salaried hospital doctors, including the best trained specialists. Younger, better-trained doctors are increasingly seeking hospital positions rather than opening up private practice clinics, even though they realize that they will earn less money. As a result, the number of clinics has been declining.

The clinic system is very different from what we see in the United States. In Japan, doctors in private practice are permitted to operate inpatient clinics with up to nineteen beds, which, by law, can be occupied for forty-eight hours or less. Since such doctors do not have hospital privileges, they compete by buying expensive technology for their clinics. As a result, Japan has more CT and MRI scanners than any other country, including the United States (23.2 MRIs scanners per million persons versus 7.6 in the United States and 84.4 CT scanners versus 13.2).[12] The hospitals, especially those associated with prestigious universities, are generally known to offer superior care; however, they do not work on the basis of appointments. So there is an inconvenience trade-off in going to a superior university clinic and waiting versus getting a specific appointment at the local doctor's clinic.

Until recently the hospitals have not been nearly as technologically sophisticated as ours, because the Japanese are not eager to spend money on technology that will not produce a good return on the investment. However, Japanese patients stay in the hospital far longer than Americans do—during the mid-1990s, our average length of stay was 5.1 days while theirs ranged from 15.8 to 29.1 days depending on the hospital. This is explained, in large part, by the fact that the Japanese have not been ready to build nursing homes for extended-stay patients. Remember, this is a traditional society where women have historically stayed home and cared for aging parents and sick relatives. More women are now working, but the health care delivery system has not yet caught up. People have dealt with the change in women's roles by checking in their elderly relatives for an extended stay when the work of caring for the aging relative gets too burdensome or when they go on vacation. The upshot of the long length of hospital stay is that other patients must wait to be admitted, even those who need urgent attention.

In the spring of 2000, the government agreed to do something about the problem. It passed legislation funding long-term care for the elderly. However, there are very few nursing homes ready to accept elderly patients, and Japanese society is not entirely prepared to institutionalize elderly relatives. The shift in attitude and behavior is expected to move forward slowly, making the transition manageable both socially and financially.

When Americans discover that Japanese patients bring their own soap, night clothes, towels, and other necessities to the hospital, including food prepared by the family, they conclude that Japanese hospitals are not nearly modern enough. Care provided by family members is becoming less typical as more women, who have traditionally provided such care, enter the workforce and have no time for such activities; however, private nurses have always been and still are a common feature. Finally, Americans find Japanese hospitals to be dingy and extremely short on privacy. For their part, the Japanese are not dissatisfied with their hospitals, which shows, once again, that understandings about comfort and essential amenities are a matter of cultural expectations.

It is also worth noting that the Japanese spend much less than we do on health care, which explains why the hospitals do not have the amenities that Americans associate with quality of care. Other factors that explain how they can spend so much less than we do begin with the fact that they have about one-third less surgery than we do—for instance, organ replacement is culturally unacceptable and restricted by law. Remember, hospital procedures, particularly surgery, are the most expensive categories of care. The Japanese also do not have our social problems, like violence and poverty, which requires expensive health care services, especially emergency room care.

When the Japanese economy slumped during the 1990s, the Japanese instituted increased control over health care costs—specifically over prices, fee schedules, and treatment volume—and implemented an increase in co-payments. This led to a decrease in health expenditures in 2002 for the first time in Japan's history. This decrease does not show up as a decline in percentage of GDP spent on health, because the GPD also contracted.[13] Economic stagnation led to increased attention to proposals for more radical reforms, including more bundling of hospital reimbursements and revision of health insurance reimbursement arrangements. There has been some talk about market-based medicine—for example, allowing the expansion of for-profit hospitals and consumer-oriented practice. The latter is in response to patient complaints about long waiting times and doctors who are unwilling to give out information. One of the reasons that doctors do not share information is that Japan's medical record keeping is not up-to-date and doctors may not have the information available to them. Changes are being introduced, but none are likely to happen very quickly, nor are they expected to be revolutionary, because of resistance from entrenched interest groups.

Are there lessons to be learned from the Japanese? Their health care system does not seem to be something we would want to emulate. However, they live longer than anyone else does in the world, and they spend less than half of what we spend. What else can you conclude but that they are doing something right beyond creating an outstanding health care delivery system? By the way, I will not let you dismiss the differences by saying that it is their diet. Yes, their diet plays a critical role; that cannot be denied. But their diet has not changed very much over the last thirty years or so, during the period when their life expectancy skyrocketed to the top of the international life-expectancy scales. It is also true that they have long led the world in the rate of stomach cancer; they smoke at an incredibly high rate; their cities have been highly polluted in the past; they are still very crowded; and they work long hours and take little time off. I leave you to ponder these inconsistencies. If you decide to explore this issue in greater detail, I recommend that you consider the answer offered by an increasing number of researchers who believe that social arrangements across social institutions have more to do with the health status of a country's inhabitants than its health care system, which as a single social institution cannot overcome factors linked to ill health that are associated with the operations of other social institutions (e.g., education or labor market).[14]

CONCLUSION

So what have we learned from this brief overview of how other people have decided to shape their health care delivery systems? One thing that seems obvious is that different societies have dealt with their concerns about health care in different ways in part because they started doing so at differing times in history. Once their foundations were in place, people simply continued construction. Retrospectively, we can see that the 1960s, the mid-1980s, and the years just before and after the turn of the twenty-first century produced some notable trends in a number of countries.

The 1960s signaled a period of post–World War II economic growth and prosperity in most countries. Having had a decade to recover from the war, countries turned their attention to internal social issues. This period is when the United States created Medicare and Medicaid and when Canada instituted universal health care coverage. By the mid- to late 1980s, virtually every industrialized country found itself confronting rising health care costs and became convinced that there was no end to it in sight. This is when U.S. policy makers and health care administrators began telling us that the competition was the single best solution to the problem. Policy makers in other countries found some of the arrangements developed in the United States worth testing. What is interesting to see is how competition appears when other countries embrace it. Somehow it does not turn out looking much as it does in this country. By the late 1990s, the United States began focusing on mechanisms designed to measure quality of care, such as new data-collection measures and trend-indicating software. Policy makers in other countries have taken an interest in these developments as well.[15]

Can we, in turn, learn from the experiences of other countries? Perhaps. You might have noticed in reading this chapter that at least one of the mechanisms we created bears a strong similarity to arrangements European countries have had in place for a long time. Consider the fact that sickness funds, which grew out of mutual-benefit societies, were built on the idea that everyone would contribute the same amount of money to maintain the fund even though they would not necessarily benefit from it during any one year, perhaps not ever. Sounds a little like the basis of the Blue Cross plan, doesn't it? Americans celebrate the founding of BC–BS as a totally new idea invented in the United States.

Americans tend toward xenophobia—we seem to have a strong need to reject what is foreign. Unlike the Europeans and Japanese, who have been importing ideas based on our experiments, we prefer to think that we are better off creating new mechanisms from scratch. And we do keep inventing a steady stream of new mechanisms to apply to health care delivery operations, which we are prepared to reject and discard when they fail to deliver what they promised. Then, we simply go on to innovate some more. Winston Churchill's judgment of American ingenuity may be apropos here. He is said to have observed that Americans can be counted on to make the right decisions—after exhausting every other possible option.

NOTES

1. Odin Anderson, *Health Care: Can There Be Equity? The United States, Sweden, and England* (New York: Wiley-Interscience, 1972).

2. Joseph White, *Competing Solutions: American Health Care Proposals and International Experience* (Washington, D.C.: Brookings Institution, 1995), 121.

3. Rudolf Klein, "Britain's National Health Service Revisited," *New England Journal of Medicine* 350 (February 26, 2004): 937–42; Peter Smith and Nick York, "Quality Incentives: The Case of U.K. General Practitioners," *Health Affairs* 23 (May/June, 2004): 112–18; Simon Stevens, "Reform Strategies for the English NHS," *Health Affairs* 23(May/June 2004): 37–44.

4. Klein, "Britain's National Health," 937.

5. Carolyn Hughes Tuohy, "Dynamics of a Changing Health Sphere: The United States, Britain, and Canada," *Health Affairs* 18 (May/June, 1999): 129.

6. Julia Abelson, Matthew Mendelsohn, John Lavis, Steven Morgan, Pierre-Gerlier Forest, and Marilyn Swinton, "Canadians Confront Health Care Reform," *Health Affairs* 23 (May/June 2004): 186–93.

7. John Iglehart, "Germany's Health Care System (First of Two Parts)," *New England Journal of Medicine* 324 (February 14, 1991): 503–8.

8. Deborah Stone, *The Limits of Professional Power* (Chicago: University of Chicago Press, 1980).

9. Reinhard Busse, "Disease Management Programs in Germany's Statutory Health Insurance System," *Health Affairs* 23 (May/June 2004): 56–67.

10. Lawrence Brown and Volker Amelung, "'Manacled Competition' Market Reforms in German Health Care," *Health Affairs* 18 (May/June 1999): 88.

11. Naoki Ikegami and John Creighton Campbell, "Health Care Reform in Japan: The Virtues of Muddling Through," *Health Affairs* 18 (May/June, 1999): 56–75; John Iglehart, "Japan's Medical Care System," *New England Journal of Medicine* 319 (September 22, 1988): 807–12.

12. Gerard Anderson, Uwe Reinhardt, Peter Hussey, and Varduhi Petrosyan, "It's the Prices, Stupid: Why the United States Is So Different from Other Countries," *Health Affairs* 22 (May/June 2003): 99.

13. Naoki Ikegami and John Creighton Campbell, "Japan's Health Care System: Containing Costs and Attempting Reform," *Health Affairs* 23 (May/June 2004): 26–36; M. G. Marmot and George Davey Smith, "Why Are the Japanese Living Longer?" *British Medical Journal* 299 (December 23/30, 1989): 1547–51.

14. Grace Budrys, *Unequal Health: How Inequality Contributes to Health or Illness* (Lanham, Md.: Rowman and Littlefield, 2003).

15. Peter Hussey, Gerard Anderson, Robin Osburn, Colin Feek, Vivienne McLaughlin, John Millar, and Arnold Epstein, "How Does the Quality of Care Compare in Five Countries?" *Health Affairs* 23 (May/June 2004): 89–99.

11

Health Care System Reform

Never before had Congress enacted major Medicare legislation about which the divisions between the political parties ran so deep. The most critical voice was that of Senator Edward M. Kennedy (D-Mass.). . . . Kennedy asked, "Who do you trust? The HMO-coddling, drug-company-loving, Medicare-destroying, Social-Security-hating Bush administration? Or do you trust Democrats who created Medicare and will fight with you to defend it every day of every week of every year?

John K. Iglehart
New England Journal of Medicine
February 19, 2004

In March 2004 the chief actuary of the Centers for Medicare & Medicaid Services revealed that as early as the previous summer, his office had esti-mated much higher costs for the proposed reforms than congressional budget analysts had. His superiors in the Bush administration, however, or-dered him to withhold the estimates from members of Congress and warned him that "the consequences for insubordination [would be] extremely se-vere." . . . Members of both parties have acknowledged that if the adminis-tration's estimates had been known to legislators and the public, significant changes would likely have been required in the final provisions of H.R. 1 [version of the Medicare Prescription Drug, Improvement, and Moderniza-tion Act of 2003 approved by the House of Representatives and passed by Congress]. . . . The concealment of budget estimates reflects the usual tug-of-war between the executive and legislative branches of government.

Thomas R. Oliver, Philip R. Lee, and Helene L. Lipton
Milbank Quarterly 82, no. 2 (2004)

The Senate task force recommended lowering health care costs through liability reforms, technology and reduced paperwork; expanding private coverage through tax credits, purchasing pools and new coverage options; and bolstering the health care safety net with new community centers, more affordable drugs and incentives for doctor participation. . . . "We have an incredible amount of evidence that incremental change doesn't work," said Georganne Chapin, president of Hudson Health Plan, a nonprofit managed care organization in Tarrytown, N.Y. . . . "Incremental programs are extraordinarily expensive, and they are by nature temporary and don't really contribute to the health security of people individually or the population at large," she said.

Markian Hawryluk
American Medical News
May 24–31, 2004

This chapter addresses health care reform. It confirms what we have found thus far, that reform is a never-ending process. Each time a new plan is proposed, even before it is enacted, the health sector participants who are most likely to be affected prepare for it by finding ways to reduce the impact of planned changes. Their resistance invariably leads to a new set of problems that produces a new wave of proposals, and so it goes. We will review the recent crop of health insurance reform proposals purporting to increase access to care. We will go on to consider critics' reactions to the proposals. As you will see, the criticisms largely revolve around concerns about the impact on costs, meaning that two of the three objectives governing the health care system (access and cost containment) have been occupying the center of attention. Since the third goal, quality, has not gotten as much attention as costs in debates about proposals aimed at increasing access, we will consider it separately.

As we saw in the last chapter, the United States is unique in the extent to which it depends on free market competition to balance the goals of cost containment, access, and quality of care. Comparing our results to those achieved by other countries, we find that

- costs are higher in the United States than in other countries;
- nearly a fifth of Americans do not have access to care while everyone in other highly advanced countries has access; and
- there is nothing to indicate that we are enjoying higher quality of care, especially considering that Americans do not live as long as people in other countries.

Clearly, the market approach failed to deliver on what its proponents promised. In light of this record, some policy makers have taken the position that moving toward greater government oversight is the only logical step to take; others continue to argue that we should try harder to make competition work. The latter have prevailed because the public is divided and political climate favors private-sector solutions. Given the record of experimentation with market forces, you should expect the following discussion to be highly critical of that approach.

HEALTH INSURANCE REFORM

New legislative proposals keep appearing because neither the majority of policy makers nor the members of the public have been ready to embrace previous attempts. The proposals may be new, but it seems that they are not particularly original. In fact, the Institute of Medicine (IOM) says that all the proposals that have been introduced in recent years fall into one of the following four categories:

- Employer mandates that require employers to provide insurance for all employees, as well as national mandates that require all others to be covered by public plans
- Individual mandates requiring everyone to buy personal insurance with the aid of tax credits
- The single-payer plan
- The incremental approach that depends on expansion of existing public programs—that is, Medicare, Medicaid, and SCHIP, often with government assistance to allow the uninsured to buy into these programs[1]

Employer and Individual Mandates

The first alternative, the employer mandate option, is the least popular option because the majority of Americans believe businesses should not be so closely regulated by the government. However, the insurance industry has come up with a plan that aims to extend insurance to one particular category of uninsured—employees of small companies that cannot afford the cost of insurance at current rates. The Association Health Plan proposal would provide a less-expensive insurance option that would also be less comprehensive and not covered by state insurance laws. Critics say that allowing this proposal to go forward would permit insurance companies to offer better plans to businesses with healthier employees and further reduce the benefits for those whose employees are at greater risk of becoming injured or sick. The Center for Health System Change calculated that small companies that do not provide insurance employ sixteen million persons.[2] It estimates that even if the government were to provide a 30 percent premium subsidy, which is of course quite high, that would result in only 1.5 million workers benefiting. Since most observers accept the validity of this assessment, the plan does not have much support from anyone outside the insurance industry.

The second option, individual mandate, requires all Americans to buy their own insurance and depend on the government's allocating funds to cover a "tax credit." The current plan proposes offering a $3,000 credit for a family of four with an income of $25,000 or less. As income goes up, the amount of the tax credit declines. As you may remember from previous discussion, the average cost of an individual plan (when purchased through an employer) is about $3,300 and about $9,000 for a family plan. Insurance coverage purchased independently varies in price and coverage to a far greater extent. Because such policies do not provide good value for the money, only 4.5 percent of Americans purchased individual plans in recent years. While tax credit plans have been touted in some quarters, critics point out that the projected tax credits do not come close to covering the cost of insurance. So the idea that a tax credit of this magnitude will give low-income, uninsured persons an incentive to purchase insurance is not convincing.

The insurance industry has had no reason to offer more attractive plans to date. However, the government gave the insurance industry a big bonus in 2003—Health Saving Accounts—which has given the industry a great deal of incentive to create a new, less-expensive plan for employed persons.

Health Savings Accounts depend on employers arranging to take money out of the employee's check, which is then set aside in a tax-free account to be used for health care. The Medicare Prescription Drug Improvement Act of 2003 (which we discussed briefly with the Medicare plan in chapter 7 and with Medicare + Choice in chapter 8) authorized $7 billion to cover the loss in tax revenues. This legislation encouraged the insurance industry to create low cost plans that carry a high deductible.

Those who oppose the "consumer-driven" approach to health care, which is how these plans are being presented, argue that the majority of people who are uninsured do not make enough money to pay taxes, so allowing them to put money into a tax free account to achieve tax savings makes no sense. More troubling, they say, is that younger, healthier employees are the ones who are most likely to opt for this alternative, which leaves those who have health problems facing higher costs and the possibility of being uninsurable. Policy makers call this "adverse selection." Critics use other labels, including "social Darwinism." Ron Pollack, the spokesman for a well-established health consumer group, Families USA, employed this label in testimony before Congress.[3] He reminded the listeners that 5 percent of the public uses about 50 percent of the health care dollar, but there is no way to predict who will fall into that 5 percent. Thus, he pointed out, this kind of plan ⬛⬛⬛ n acceptance of a "every man for himself" philosophy.

To give further support to the consumer-driven health agenda, th ⬛⬛⬛ e Prescription Drug Act includes a provision establishing pilot projects in a number of as yet unnamed cities by the year 2010 where direct competition between Medicare and private plans would be inaugurated, a scenario generally referred to as *privatization*. Critics say is this is a direct attack on the essence of public insurance as we have known it.

The Single-Payer Plan

The third alternative identified by the IOM is the single-payer plan. The most recent version is the one presented by the Physicians' Working Group for Single-Payer National Health Insurance in a 2003 article in the *Journal of the American Medical Association*.[4] The proposal is based on four principles:

- Insurance coverage should not be tied to employment.
- The right to choose a physician is fundamental.
- Corporate profit has no place in caregiving.
- Medical decisions should be determined by patients and doctors, not corporations or government bureaucrats.

The authors say that "the United States alone treats health care as a commodity distributed according to the ability to pay, rather than as a social service to be distributed according to medical need."[5] They argue that the advantages of providing universal access are obvious—an enormous number of lives would be saved. People would also be healthier, therefore more productive. Furthermore, they would not run up high costs that result from delayed care. Others have pointed out that half the country's bankruptcies are due at least in part to medical debt, which means that those persons likely delay care because they can no longer afford it and are sure to run up high costs when they are finally forced to seek care.

The authors of the single-payer proposal maintain that eliminating private insurance would result in an immediate drop in health care expenditures because administrative costs would decline sharply. They point out that private health insurance consumes 12 percent of premiums on average, whereas Medicare consumes about 3 percent. In fact, two of the authors of the single-payer plan article argue elsewhere that the government's health care cost burden is currently being underestimated. They say that the only costs being considered are direct government expenditures on Medicare, Medicaid, Veterans Administration, public health, and hospital subsidies. They argue that tax subsidies that the government extends to employers for offering insurance and expenditures on public employee health insurance costs should be included. This more accurate calculation, they say, raises the government share of health care costs to 59.8 percent rather than the 45.3 percent the government reports.[6] Thus, they say that the government's contribution is actually a matter of "public funding" plus "tax financing." In short, they advocate eliminating this tax loss and using the additional funds this would produce to fund a national health care plan. Another way of looking at it is that we are already spending nearly as much as countries that have national health programs.

Two economists, Jack Hadley and John Holahan, published what has become a widely quoted assessment of how much it would cost to provide universal coverage.[7] They argue that universal coverage would not increase costs as much as opponents have said because the money being spent to cover the costs of caring for the uninsured and underinsured are not generally figured into universal coverage projections. They estimate that the uninsured received approximately $98.9 billion in care in 2001, of which $34.5 billion was uncompensated. Uncompensated care is not "free," since somebody has to pay for it. Most of it is paid for by the government either through subsidized Medicare and Medicaid payments or state and local government taxes. They admit that universal coverage would cause some people to use more services than they do now but that it would probably not be much more than what is being used by those who are currently covered. Using that kind of logic, the two researchers calculated that universal coverage would cost $33.9 billion to $68.7 billion in 2001 dollars, which amounts to an increase of 3 percent to 6 percent and would translate, at most, into less than a 1 percent increase in percentage of GDP we spend on health.

Yet another source of funding has been identified by analysts associated with the IOM, who estimate that the economic losses stemming from lack of health insurance amounts to $65 billion to $130 billion a year due to higher disease and death rates among the uninsured.[8] They argue that there would be no increased cost, since the rate of economic loss due to people not working to their full capacity is higher than the estimated cost of providing insurance for all Americans.

One of the main objections opponents of the single-payer plan bring up is that increased control on the part of the government will have a negative impact on the expansion of technology. Those who take the opposite stance counter with the observation that while it is true that the United States employs more technology than many other countries, there is no consistent pattern of technological expansion across countries and no clear link between expansion on technology and the total national expenditure on health.[9] The evidence on Japan's expenditure profile is often used to illustrate this point. As you will recall from the last chapter, Japan has the most technology and spends a smaller proportion of its GDP on health than do most other countries.

Another objection is that people should be able to buy more and better care if they are willing to pay for it. A number of analysts who favor universal coverage concur, concluding that allowing a two-tier system of care to develop may be the only way that the United States will ever accept a national health plan.

Incremental Reform

The debate on universal coverage may have brought in an increasing number of researchers armed with stacks of data to the table, but that has done little to sway the public. As you may recall from chapter 3, the public has been more concerned about terrorism and the economy than health care issues since September 11. As long as that continues to be true, policy experts do not expect the country to move to a more bold type of reform.[10] That leaves the fourth alternative outlined by the IOM, incremental reform, which is exactly how we have been addressing health care reform in recent years.[11] Various pieces of legislation aimed at extending Medicare, Medicaid, and SCHIP have been enacted. The problem is that these legislative reforms have not succeeded in extending health insurance to many more Americans, which means that we can expect to see a steady stream of new reform proposals up for debate in the foreseeable future.

PRESCRIPTION DRUG LEGISLATION AND PHARMACEUTICAL COSTS

The fact that we as a society have opted for incremental reform should not be taken to mean that the reform agenda has become any less contentious than it was during the early 1990s, when radical reform was being debated. Far from it! To illustrate the point, we need to return to the Medicare Prescription Drug, Improvement, and Modernization Act of 2003, a 678-page bill, which some legislators readily admitted they did not read in full. As you already know, it includes a variety of provisions, including support for Health Savings Accounts. At this point, we will focus on the main thrust of the bill, which is designed to provide drug coverage to Medicare enrollees beginning in 2006.

The law instituted a drug discount card, which Medicare enrollees may purchase for $30. It also provided a $600 drug subsidy for low-income enrollees.

The biggest problem with the legislation according to critics is its complexity. The plan requires a person to pay a deductible of $250 per year and a premium of $35 per month. It is, however, the "doughnut hole" that has attracted the greatest amount of criticism. The plan pays 75 percent of the cost up to $2,250, after which it pays nothing until drug expenses go up to $5,100. This gap is the doughnut hole. Once a person spends $5,100, the person pays 5 percent for all additional drug costs for the remainder of the year. What this means is that some beneficiaries will be shocked to find that they must spend more than they spent before the so-called drug benefit went into effect. Consider the following examples:

> A relatively healthy 65-year old man with hypertension who now spends $730 per year filling his brand-name prescription at his local pharmacy would spend a total of $790 per year, including premiums ($420), the deductible ($250), and coinsurance. Thus, he would spend more in premiums and cost sharing than his drugs actually cost. During the same year, a 79-year-old woman with multiple chronic (but common) conditions, including a history of congestive heart failure, hypertension, chronic arthritic pain, and Parkinson's disease, who takes nine different generic and brand name medicines costing about $4,600 per year would pay $3,520 in premiums, deductibles, and cost sharing; she would fall into the doughnut hole.[12]

It is easy to identify the basic problem here—namely, the high cost of drugs. The question of why drugs cost so much has been receiving a great deal of attention. Prescription drug spending has been the fastest growing component of the health care bill over the last couple of decades, for which there are a number of reasons. One is that more patients are developing chronic illnesses that can be treated with drugs. Another reason, one that has been true all along but has now been written into law, is the clause in the 2003 drug bill specifically prohibiting Medicare from engaging in negotiations over drug prices. Governments in all other industrialized countries negotiate over drug prices with drug manufacturers. Indeed, according to one group of analysts, the doughnut hole could be eliminated if Medicare could negotiate and achieve prices similar to those paid by citizens in Canada, France, and the United Kingdom.[13] It is also interesting to note that no one seems to mind that the Veterans Administration and major health plans in this country have been negotiating prices all along and that they pay far less than the rest of us for the drugs they buy.

The biggest reason that explains why drugs constitute the high proportion of the health budget, according to many observers including the U.S. Government Accountability Office (GAO), is "direct-to-consumer" advertising. As we can all attest, there has been an explosion of television, magazine, and Internet drug ads over the last few years. People are advised to "ask your doctor" about drugs for conditions that are not always identified but come with the assurance that we will feel much better after taking them.

Drug companies say that they are providing a valuable service by informing people about symptoms they need to check out. The companies also maintain that they need to increase their profits so that they can support research and development (R&D) of new drugs. Critics have a lot to say about both claims. One particularly harsh critic, Dr. Marcia Angell, former editor of the *New England Journal of Medicine*, presents a scathing analysis of a whole range of claims made by the pharmaceutical industry.[14] She calculates that R&D amounts to about 11 to 14 percent of sales while "marketing and administration" amounts to about 36 percent. She notes that accurate numbers are hard to get because the industry includes what it calls "education," legal fees, and executive salaries, as well as promotion and advertising, in the marketing and administration category. She is not alone in noting that research is often funded by the National Institutes of Health and other agencies that support clinical trials involving new forms of treatment. In other words, some pharmaceutical R&D is supported by tax dollars.

A recent *New York Times* story casts additional light on where some of the "marketing and administration" money might be going.[15] It seems that drug companies have been sending unsolicited checks of $10,000 to doctors, inviting them to serve as "consultants." The only thing the attached consulting agreement requires is agreement to prescribe the company's medicines, with no reporting requirement. The story says that the doctors being interviewed were sending the checks back.

Even more surprising is Angell's contention that pharmaceutical R&D activities result in far less innovation than the drug companies would like us to believe. Angell says that instead of coming up with new drugs, drug companies are actually reformulating old drugs, which she calls "me-too" drugs. They change a minor component in existing drugs to seek a new patent to protect their rights to the formula for the next fourteen years. (Congress extended patent coverage from eight years to fourteen years in 2000.) Then the drug companies proceed to give the reformulated drug a new name and market it as a new and far more effective drug. Other analysts say that not only have drug companies concentrated their efforts on producing me-too drugs and lifestyle drugs but that they are failing to produce drugs that would be more socially beneficial. They are not focusing their efforts on producing drugs for common chronic diseases, emerging diseases, and potential bioterrorism threats.[16]

Angell also tells us that "of the seventy-eight new drugs approved by the FDA in 2002, only seventeen contained new active ingredients, and only seven of these were classified by the FDA as improvements over older drugs."[17] None of the seven came from a major U.S. drug company. Americans have been led to believe that American drug companies alone can be trusted to produce drugs safely. However, half the largest drug companies, which produce the most commonly used drugs, are based in Europe, and the drugs are manufactured all over the world, which makes one wonder why there has been so much talk about the risks associated with "reinportation" of drugs. Winning the legislative battle to reinport drugs from Canada may be satisfying to some, but it is obviously not an impressive national policy solution. Meanwhile, because the United States offers such great moneymaking opportunities, Internet pharmacies have come into existence, some of which are untrustworthy.[18]

HEALTH CARE SCAMS

If you are beginning to get the idea that the health industry is so lucrative that those who might be willing to engage in shady practices will find ways to take advantage, you are exactly right. What is more troubling is that major health care corporations are engaging in big-time fraud. Angell says that there has been a "litany of charges" against pharmaceutical companies, including overcharging Medicare and Medicaid, colluding with generic companies to keep generic drugs off the market, illegally promoting drugs for unapproved uses, engaging in misleading advertising, and so forth. They have also been found covering up findings, which they do by preventing negative findings from being published by the clinical researchers whose investigations they support.[19]

According to the Justice Department, federal officials recouped $1.7 billion from health care companies under the False Claims Act in 2003.[20] The False Claims Act (commonly known as the Sarbanes-Oxley Act) was passed in 2002 in response to the corporate scandals at Enron, Arthur Andersen, and others. The act allows whistleblowers to receive a share of what the government recovers, which is now recovering thirteen dollars for every one dollar it spends on enforcement. Four of the ten largest settlements in 2003 involve health care companies: Health Corporation of America for $631 million; and three pharmaceutical companies, Abbott Labs, AstraZeneca, and Bayer Corporation, which each settled for between $250 and $400 million.

As if that were not enough, bad actors involved in health insurance scams seemingly appeared out of nowhere and succeeded in duping more than two hundred thousand policyholders and fifteen thousand employers between 2000 and 2002. According to the GAO, the Department of Labor identified 144 entities not authorized to sell insurance with the result of leaving policyholders with $252 million in unpaid medical claims.[21]

There is no question that corporate crime and fraud has been rampant in this country. It is just that most people believe that defrauding people who are ill or at risk of becoming ill to be especially reprehensible. Why this is happening is not so mysterious according to some observers. The answer is either too much competition or too little competition, depending on the perspective from which one views the situation.

Too Much Competition or Too Little?

Taking the "too-little" side of the argument, the American Medical Association (AMA) claims that the problem is that megacorporations have too much power. When corporations become very large, they become less interested in lowering their prices to compete with other companies. The AMA argues that this ultimately leads to corporate malfeasance, but it does not say why. It may not "want to go there" to explain. Some observers argue that the source of the problem is that various industries, including the doctors' lobby, are giving so much money to politicians that they are virtually buying favorable legislation and protection from legislation that might stem some of the malfeasance.

Doctors and Antitrust

As an aside, I should note that the AMA's main concern is that doctors are not permitted to negotiate over prices, because they are defined as small businesspersons or independent contractors by law. Engaging in negotiations over prices is strictly prohibited under antitrust law. It is their negotiating position vis-à-vis insurance companies, health plans, and HMOs that doctors want to be made more favorable. That has been a difficult struggle because Congress fears that allowing doctors to negotiate will open the door for a whole range of occupational groups to demand the same right to which the business community objects vigorously. The complication from the doctors' perspective is that insurance companies are not regulated by the federal government, thanks to the McCarran Ferguson Act of 1945, which declared insurance to be something other than a business and exempted the insurance industry from oversight by the federal government.

There is more to this story. The federal government gave the states the right to regulate insurance companies. However, corporations that employ five hundred persons and have set aside funds to cover insurance (i.e., have self-insured) can also avoid state regulation based on a 1974 piece of legislation, the Employee Retirement Income Security Act (ERISA). What this means is that they can offer as much or as little coverage as they like and cut off benefits for certain kinds of care—costly chronic illnesses, for example. This practice is defined as discriminatory and prohibited by state insurance laws when it is done by independent insurance companies. In recent years, the courts have begun to set more rigid restrictions on the interpretation of ERISA as an increasing number of challenges have come before the courts. However, in 2004 the Supreme Court determined that ERISA preempts law suits against managed care organizations. It will be interesting to see how conflict over what this law is supposed to achieve plays out.

Blue Cross–Blue Shield conversions

The AMA has a lot of company in opposing the trend toward the development of megacorporations. One of the most topical illustrations involves the recent wave of BC–BS conversions from nonprofit to for-profit status followed by mergers to form much larger corporations. Political leaders and consumer groups across the country have been opposed to the conversions. Where deals have been struck—between BC–BS and the state of New York, for example—the politicians were satisfied, but consumer groups were not. New York allowed the conversion to go through in exchange for an agreement to direct the funds from the sale into state coffers. Opponents argued that the funds should go to supporting nonprofit organizations rather than to subsidizing the state budget. In other cases, conversions and/or mergers with for-profit health plans have been opposed because BC–BS administrators arranged to get a huge bonus out of the deal. That was true in Washington state, where the CEO was scheduled to get $2.2 million out of the deal.[22] However, because the objections to this and other conversions were so widely publicized and because they produced a groundswell of feeling on the part of consumers, politicians have made it clear that conversions would no longer be permitted. No new Blues conversion plans were announced in 2004.

Why the BC–BS plans were so eager to convert is worth considering more closely. Some business analysts say that the BC–BSs that did convert have been no more profitable than the ones that continue as nonprofits. There is also general agreement that the only way the newly converted operations can be more profitable is by raising rates. If conversion and consolidation do not increase profits or reduce prices, what effect does it have? Most observers agree that it makes the newly formed companies bigger and more powerful, and that is exactly what has the critics so upset. Being more powerful allows the insurance companies or health plans to set prices without engaging in much negotiation. Being as large as they are allows them to walk away from deals with doctors, hospitals, and employers, which are all far smaller in size, without risking much loss of income.

Health Sector Competition

Then there is the "too-much" side of the competition debate. Here we find those who claim that the emphasis on competition has encouraged participants to come up with new business ventures that have no social benefit and are in fact pushing the legal limits. To illustrate, the health sector has witnessed the emergence of problems associated with self-referral to doctor-owned clinics, specialty hospitals, and "boutique medicine."

With the growth of HMOs and tighter controls on reimbursements, doctors stepped up their efforts to gain a larger share of the health care dollar by building clinics equipped with the latest and most expensive technology. Then they proceeded to refer patients to the clinics they owned for tests rather than to the hospital laboratories they had been using. The hospitals were not pleased. Suits and countersuits mounted. The Centers for Medicare and Medicaid Services eventually got involved, setting forth regulations on when it would consider such referrals to be legitimate and reimbursable.

The competitive environment is also credited for the emergence of "specialty hospitals." Doctors, sometimes alone and sometimes with financial backers, decided that competition combined with other business strategies provided an excellent model for creating a "focused-factory" approach to treatment, with the aim of increasing productivity and reducing costs. By the end of 2003, there were one hundred specialty hospitals in existence across the country, most focusing on cardiac, orthopedic, surgical procedures, and women's health. Twenty-six more hospitals were in the process of development before the Centers for Medicare and Medicaid Services announced a moratorium on physician investment and referrals to specialty hospitals. The ban was written into law as part of the Medicare Prescription Drug, Improvement, and Modernization Act of 2003, in response to a major study conducted by the GAO of the consequences for the entire U.S. health care system.[23]

In the meantime, a small number of doctors have come up with yet another innovation. They have begun offering middle-class patients (read: patients who are able to afford it) "boutique" or "concierge" services for a fixed fee. The idea is that patients can pay, let's say $99 per month, for which they might receive twenty-four-hour cell phone and e-mail access, same-day appointments, routine checkups and preventive medicine not generally covered by insurance, house calls, wellness programs, and nutrition counseling.

What is the problem with boutique medicine, you might ask? If people want that and can afford it, shouldn't they be able to buy it? One reason is that Medicare rules prohibit it. To participate in Medicare, which almost all doctors do, they must agree not to charge extra fees and may be legally liable if they do so. Physicians, especially those who care for the poor, object to such practices because they primarily function to divide the haves from the have-nots, which they say is unethical. Beyond that, they say, such practices add to the overall cost of health care without providing any wider social benefit.

THEORETICAL ARGUMENTS FOR AND AGAINST COMPETITION

Are you beginning to see theoretical perspectives coming into play here? In this case, the argument is between those who favor the explanation espoused by economists who belong to the classical school of economics and economists who argue that the health care sector is a special case and does not fit the classical model. This argument has been going on for quite some time, and there is some parallel here with the debate between the functionalists and conflict theorists in sociology.[24] The difference, however, is that classical economists are far more assertive than sociologists in arguing that "free market" competition is the best arrangement for the distribution of all goods and services. Economists on the other side of this debate carry no label, but their position is comparable to that of the conflict theorists in sociology. The economists who disagree with the classical school of economics argue that health care must be treated as a special case and an exception to the classical model. They generally begin by referring to a 1963 article by Kenneth Arrow, a Nobel Prize–winning economist who outlined the reasons for looking at health care that way.[25]

The position taken by classical economists is that there is an "invisible hand" controlling the distribution of all goods and services, including health care services, under free market conditions, ensuring that a sufficient supply of X will be produced to match the demand for X. Ideal market conditions are characterized by the following:

- Many sellers and many buyers, resulting in steady, ongoing competition
- Easy entry of new firms and exit of firms that fail
- Excellent information for comparative shopping
- High responsiveness to pricing, reflecting consumer preference
- Constant innovation resulting in increasing value

Opponents say that the health market is characterized by the following:

- The product is difficult to evaluate and, in some cases, may be so new that it still does not have a performance record.
- The seller (the physician) is the buyer's agent, controls information and moment of decision; moreover, buyers want it that way.

- Shopping is costly and complex, not a sensible approach if other alternatives are available.
- Medical services are not a product most people want to purchase, so the incentives are different.
- "Utility theory" is difficult to satisfy, meaning that a person's priorities are clear; the benefits and risks are fully known; and most important, the buyer can order all of this information to make a rational choice.

Proponents and opponents of market solutions agree that the U.S. experiment with health sector competition has failed to control costs. Health care costs have risen to a greater extent in this country than they have in other industrialized nations since the 1980s, when it first began this experiment. No factors that are currently adding to the cost of health care can explain that trend. Many other countries have more health personnel, more doctor visits, and a greater proportion of aged and chronically ill than we do. Critics of our health care arrangements say that our costs are higher because the purchasers of services are highly fragmented and have little bargaining power, which constitutes the main difference between the United States and other countries. In other countries, the single buyer or a small number of buyers have a great deal of power to demand lower prices. In the United States, by contrast, suppliers of health goods and services are in a position to set high prices without having to bargain with the buyers.

Proponents and critics agree that the free market operates on the principle of *caveat emptor,* which translates into "buyer beware." However, they interpret the advantages and disadvantages differently. Proponents say that it makes buyers more sensitive to cost and prevents *moral hazard,* a term economists use to capture the idea that many of us cannot resist the temptation to use products and services that are free even if we do not need them. Those who are opposed to reliance on competition in the health sector say that *caveat emptor* is the wrong principle on which to base health care arrangements. Opponents have also been saying that competition does not increase efficiency and reduce costs. Instead, competition produces inefficiencies by creating instability, which happens when established and familiar organizations are sold or merged. Those transitions bring new faces and new rules, and that is what reduces efficiency as the new organizations become established, adopt new procedures, shift personnel, and so on. A competitive environment does encourage beneficial innovation. The problem is that it also encourages negative innovation—that is, the development of fraudulent products and services. It encourages testing the limits of legality, which is, of course, why the *caveat emptor* warning exists. The prevention of shady practices and outright fraud requires a great deal of costly monitoring and explains, in part, why the administrative costs are so much higher under competitive arrangements than they are under noncompetitive arrangements like the arrangements that exist in other countries.

HEALTH CARE QUALITY

So far we have been discussing changes in our health care arrangements that have been proposed for the primary purpose of reducing costs while achieving increased access. We have not devoted much attention to efforts aimed at addressing quality. The topic has been receiving a separate but steady stream of commentary, mostly from policy analysts plus a number of high-status members of the medical profession. The development of quality measures, the "report cards" that we discussed in chapter 7, has become a major enterprise. Coalitions including persons from leadership positions in business, medicine, and policy analysis emerge from time to time to form organizations for the specific purposes of developing better measurement instruments and setting standards of care.

Why would measuring quality be at issue now? Hasn't this been happening all along? After all, Hippocrates, the father of medicine, advocated developing a scientific basis of medical practice around 400 BC. One could argue that there has been no opposition to the idea in principle ever since (admittedly, there were all those centuries during the Middle Ages, when scientific pursuits were considered heretical). The point I want to make is that measuring quality may be popular in principle; however, in practice, it is very difficult to do.

There are three ways to think about measuring the quality of care—namely, structure, process, and outcome. Structural measures have been around the longest. Such measures focus on anything that you can count—things such as the number of fire extinguishers, width of doorways, as well as the number of physicians on staff who are board certified or the ratio of nurses to patients. While these indicators, as they applied to health care, offered clear points of comparison, most clearly applied to hospitals, critics noted that none of these measures said anything directly about the quality of care patients were receiving. That led to process measures. Measuring the process of care involves taking a sample of medical files and reviewing the entire course of medical care the patient has received. At first, the process approach was enthusiastically embraced. However, it did not take long for critics to note that the highest quality of care in the world would do no good if the initial diagnosis was incorrect.

That brought us to outcome measures based on clinical trials. The standard procedure involves assembling patients with the identical problem; sorting them according to personal characteristics — that is, sex, age, race, and insurance status (and more often these days, income and education); and randomly assigning matched pairs or categories to separate groups, with one receiving the treatment and the other not. Ideally, neither the doctor nor the patient knows whether any particular patient is receiving the treatment. This is called a *double-blind study* (both doctors and patients are blind to who is being selected to receive treatment). Identical treatment procedures are used, followed, and reported. The results are analyzed to determine if and/or how much those who received the treatment benefited.

This approach is not problem free. There are a number of serious obstacles to overcome: one, the process of doing research is expensive and time-consuming; two, it raises ethical questions about those who are being denied treatment. It is often difficult to translate positive results into practice because the cost of medications are prohibitively expensive; there are undesirable side effects that patients find objectionable; and there is no way to predict future side effects. Additionally, finding that particular procedures are ineffective does not mean that doctors will stop offering them. In fact, some may dispute the results. They may even be displeased enough to retaliate. A particularly contentious example relates to the research on treatment of back pain. The research was supported by the government-sponsored Agency for Health Care Policy and Research, which identified ten common health problems to study. It seems that early research results showed that surgery was not the best remedy, which angered the surgeons who do back surgery. They campaigned to have the agency put out of business, and they almost succeeded. However, after a couple of years of battle, the agency was renamed Agency for Healthcare Research and Quality and had its funding restored by Congress. It is now back on track and continuing to fund research for, among other things, treatment for back pain, which, by the way, additional research found to be highly effective in certain cases.

This saga focuses attention on the difficulty of translating findings into practice, an approach labeled *evidence-based medicine*. A considerable amount of work has been done on understanding when doctors change their treatment patterns and when they resist.[26] Most, not all, doctors are conservative about these things. They prefer to wait until the approach has been used in the leading medical centers by the most respected doctors in their circle and so on. Using monetary incentives — paying them more to do it — does not work nearly as well as most of us might expect. The majority of doctors really do have to be convinced that whatever is being introduced does work better. Education appears to be the best mechanism but involves a lot of time for additional training. Making the time to attend sessions for additional training, as often as it has to be done in a field that is as fast moving as medicine, is particularly challenging.

Other obvious reasons to explain why research on quality factors does not result in improvements is that it invariably raises costs, threatens established interests, and identifies problems that the health sector has been trying to resolve for a long time. The last point is illustrated by the findings on nurse staffing discussed in chapter 5. As you already know, there is a growing body of evidence showing that quality of care is better when it is provided by registered nurses. A recent study determined that registered nurses who work for more than 12.5 hours at a stretch are more likely to make mistakes but that nurses often work that many hours or more.[27] The solution is seemingly obvious—hire more nurses. However, that is exactly the problem that has proved so difficult to overcome.

Research on the number of medical specialists the country needs is another topic that has a long history. More often than not, the conclusion has been that we have too many specialists and not enough family practitioners. Researchers have consistently found that specialists employ more costly procedures. Some have argued that this may be justifiable because they provide superior care, while others say that specialists' reliance on more technology results in less-effective care.[28]

The focus on high-tech medicine is closely connected to the criticism expressed by researchers who see our health problems from a public health perspective. They argue that the attention is misdirected to treatments focusing on prolonging survival and preventing further complications of disease. They would prefer that society and the whole health research agenda shift from treating disease to preventing it. They maintain that increased attention to prevention of disease would do far more to reduce mortality from the most prevalent diseases, including heart disease and cancer, than would all the effort being devoted to studying treatment after the patient already has the disease. Americans, doctors and patients alike, do not dispute the logic of this argument. It is just that most Americans are even more interested in making sure that there will be effective treatments if and when they need them. Spending on public health has consistently remained at about 3 percent of the total health care budget. The threat of bioterrorism may produce a small increase but not nearly enough to make a major impact.

REFORM AT THE STATE LEVEL

Reform at the national level has been difficult to achieve; however, various reform measures are regularly enacted all across the country at the state level. Policy makers say that the states are individual laboratories where the search for creative solutions is less restrained. That is true. The problem is that the

plans are so different from state to state that it does not encourage one to expect that a national consensus on a single approach will be forthcoming. So
what's wrong with that? The people in those states get what they think is best
for them. Isn't that the way it should be?

Critics, no matter where they stand on the political spectrum, agree that this
is not an ideal situation for companies that have branches in more than one
state. It is difficult to coordinate health benefits for employees from one lo-
cation to another, and, as we already know, administering multiple plans is
more expensive than administering one. This raises health care costs in general and the cost of doing business in particular. That in turn makes U.S. companies less competitive, a situation businesses have been addressing by shifting a greater burden of cost to the employee, dropping coverage for the
employee's family, and hiring more workers on a part-time or short-term contract basis without health benefits.

The fact that the benefits associated with Medicaid and SCHIP are largely
determined by states is another matter that comes up in Congress on a regular basis. That issue has brought new federal mandates in the past, generally
with no additional funding. State governments must then alter the regulations
governing what is covered, and they must find the money to pay for the additional costs. Governors are unanimous in complaining about the burdens
such mandates impose. Some congressional legislators agree and have begun
to work on a major review of Medicaid.

THE INTERNET AS A PATIENT RESOURCE

There has been an explosion of health care information on the Internet. Sites
run the gamut from those created by large mainstream organizations, to individuals marketing unusual products and services that promise to bring about
spectacular changes, and to others who warn anyone who will listen about the
failures of whatever treatment they believe has failed them, and . . . there is
no end in sight. Is this explosion of health care information and advice a good
thing? Does it demystify health care treatment and make it more accessible to
patients? Or is it dangerous because it could lead some people to turn away
from legitimate health care services and get taken in by someone out to make
a quick buck or someone crazy with a grudge against doctors?

Then there is the issue of how mainstream doctors are responding to patients who come in armed with the latest information that they have found
while surfing the Internet. When a doctor discounts the patient's newfound
knowledge and expertise—is it that the doctor is just not keeping up with the
latest information, or should we put our trust in the doctor when he or she

says that the information does not apply in the patient's case? How does one tell the difference? What should doctors be doing to convince patients?

According to a 2004 survey, only 3 percent of Internet users have taken advantage of the opportunity to consult with their doctors online.[29] There are a number of hurdles to overcome. Patients say they are interested in online consultation, but they are not willing to pay much for it. Most doctors have not expressed interest in online consultation for a number of obvious reasons. Giving advice without seeing the patient has never been advisable both because the patient may be sicker than the patient realizes and the patient may turn around and sue the doctor for misdiagnosing the problem. Additionally, there is the problem of confidentiality. There are laws governing confidentiality of patient records that make using the Internet particularly risky, were a hacker to get hold of such records. The doctors who do respond via e-mail say that it works well with patients whom they have treated for a long time and whose problems they are familiar with. Whether mechanisms come into existence that make the use of doctor–patient e-mail consultations less risky remains to be seen.

CONCLUSION

Given the record of health care reform since the 1990s, most thoughtful observers have concluded that we can expect to see incremental changes in our health care delivery system rather than a major reform of the system in the foreseeable future. At the same time, that health care costs—especially out-of-pocket costs—are expected to increase means that (1) policy makers will continue to propose reforms aimed at controlling costs and (2) the public will continue to demand action regarding the cost of individual health care but not necessarily what the country as a whole pays for. Another contingent of policy makers, those most interested in quality issues, will undoubtedly continue to argue that identifying the most effective treatments while eliminating ineffective treatments and reducing medical error will improve quality and cut costs. Because recent reforms—most notably, the Medicare drug legislation—are expected to cost considerably more than initially projected, it is also possible that support for more radical reform will build up again as it did during the early 1990s.

I predict that there will be enough pressure for reform when a sufficiently large number of Americans decide to define the situation as a crisis. However, there is no way to predict exactly when that will happen. As you may recall from the discussion in chapter 2, it is not the situation itself that determines whether something is a crisis or not. It is the "definition of the situation" that determines it. In this case, society's view of our health care arrangements depends on its "construction of reality" of how serious the situation is. Undoubtedly, the health care crisis will be viewed in the larger context of life in the United States—that is, in light of concerns about homeland security. How high we put such issues as terrorism and defense as opposed to health care on the national agenda will determine whether we invest the energy required to achieve a major overhaul of the U.S. health care system or whether we can expect to hear more about proposals designed to achieve incremental reform.

NOTES

1. Institute of Medicine, *Insuring America's Health: Principles and Recommendations* (Washington, D.C.: National Academies Press, 2004).

2. Geri Aston, "Business Tax Credits Give Scant Help to Uninsured," *American Medical News* (January 14, 2002): 12.

3. Ronald Pollack, testimony at the hearing on covering the uninsured, before the Democratic Policy Committee, United States Senate, January 6, 2004.

4. The Physicians' Working Group for Single-Payer National Health Insurance, "Proposal of the Physicians' Working Group for Single-Payer National Health Insurance," *Journal of the American Medical Association* 290 (August 13): 798–805.

5. Physicians Working Group, "Proposal," 798.

6. Steffie Woolhandler and David Himmelstein, "Paying for National Health Insurance—and Not Getting It," *Health Affairs* 21 (July/August 2002): 88–98.

7. Jack Hadley and John Holahan, "Covering the Uninsured: How Much Would It Cost?" *Health Affairs* (June 4, 2003): 250–65.

8. Wilhelmine Miller, Elizabeth Richardson Vigdor, and Willard Manning, "Covering the Uninsured: What Is It Worth?" *Health Affairs* (March 31, 2004): 157–67.

9. Gerard Anderson, Uwe Reinhardt, Peter Hussey, and Varduhi Petrosyan, "It's the Prices, Stupid: Why the United States Is So Different from Other Countries," *Health Affairs* 22 (May/June 2003): 89–105.

10. Robert Blendon, John Benson, and Catherine DesRoches, "Americans' Views of the Uninsured: An Era for Hybrid Proposals," *Health Affairs* (October 23, 2003): 376–90.

11. Uwe Reinhardt, "Is There Hope for the Uninsured?" *Health Affairs* (October 23, 2003): 405–14.

12. Drew Altman, "The New Medicare Prescription-Drug Legislation," *New England Journal of Medicine* 350 (January 1, 2004): 9–10.

13. Gerard Anderson, Dennis Shea, Peter Hussey, Salomeh Keyhani, and Laurie Zephyrin, "Doughnut Holes and Price Controls," *Health Affairs* (July 21, 2004): 396–404.

14. Marcia Angell, "The Truth about the Drug Companies," *New York Review of Books* 12 (July 15, 2004): 52–58.

15. Gardiner Harris, "As Doctors Write Prescriptions, Drug Companies Write Checks," *New York Times,* June 27, 2004, 1, 19.

16. Thomas Croghan and Patricia Pittman, "The Medicine Cabinet: What's in It, Why, and Can We Change the Contents?" *Health Affairs* 23 (January/February 2004): 23–33.

17. Angell, "Truth," 56.

18. United States Government Accountability Office, "Internet Pharmacies: Some Pose Safety Risks for Consumers," June 17, 2004, GAO-04-820.

19. Tanya Albert, "Lawsuit Claims Glaxo Hid Paxil Findings," *American Medical News* (June 28, 2004): 5–6.

20. Markian Hawryluk, "Health Care Now Prime Target of Federal False Claims Act," *American Medical News* (May 10, 2004): 5–6.

21. United States Government Accountability Office, "Unauthorized or Bogus Entities Have Exploited Employers and Individuals Seeking Affordable Coverage," March 3, 2004, GAO-04–512T.

22. James Robinson, "For-Profit Non-conversion and Regulatory Firestorm at CareFirst BlueCross BlueShield," *Health Affairs* 23 (July/August 2004): 68–83; Robert Kazel, "Blues Execs to Get Bonus in Conversion," *American Medical News* (March 15, 2004): 13, 15.

23. United States Government Accountability Office, "Specialty Hospitals," October 2003, GAO-04-167.

24. Donald Light, "The Sociological Character of Health-Care Markets," *Handbook of Social Studies in Health and Medicine,* ed. Gary Albrecht, Ray Fitzpatrick, and Susan Scrimshaw (London: Sage, 2000), 394–408.

25. Kenneth Arrow, "Uncertainty and the Welfare Economics of Medical Care," *American Economic Review* 53 (December 1963): 941–73.

26. John Eisenberg, *Doctors' Decisions and the Cost of Medical Care* (Ann Arbor, Mich.: Health Administration Press, 1986).

27. Ann Rogers, Wei-Ting Hwang, Linda Scott, Linda Aiken, and David Dinges, "The Working Hours of Hospital Nurses and Patient Safety," *Health Affairs* 23 (July/August 2004): 202–12.

28. Katerine Baicker and Amitabh Chandra, "Medicare Spending, the Physician Workforce, and Beneficiaries' Quality of Care," *Health Affairs* web exclusive (April 7, 2004): 184–97.

29. Tyler Chin, "Online Consultation Slow to Grow," *American Medical News* (July 12, 2004): 1, 4.

12

The End of the Story and Its Implications

It is occasionally suggested that advances in technology can lead to reduced spending, and that may be the case in some instances. Vaccinations, for example, may sometimes offer the potential for savings, and certain types of preventive medical care may help some patients avoid costly acute care hospitalizations. But, overall, examples of new therapies for which long-term savings have been clearly demonstrated are few. Improvements in medical care that decrease mortality by helping patients avoid or survive acute health problems paradoxically increase overall spending on health care, as those (surviving) patients live to utilize health services through old age.

Douglas Holtz-Eakin
Director of the Congressional Budget Office
Testimony before the Committee on
Health, Education, Labor, and Pensions
United States Senate
January 28, 2004

What a difference two years can make. In June of 2002, physicians and patients were applauding a U.S. Supreme Court ruling upholding an Illinois law that created an independent review system for cases in which a treating physician and a patient's health plan disagree on what is medically necessary for the patient. . . . Last month the high court struck down a landmark Texas law . . . that allowed patient to sue their health plans in a state court for damages incurred when plans refused to pay for doctor-recommended treatments.

Editorial
American Medical News
July 19, 2004

This chapter signals the end of the story of how the health care delivery system in this country came to look the way it does. It is, of course, only a provisional ending, since the story continues to unfold. As a result, any conclusions we might reach are at risk of being only fleetingly accurate and temporarily applicable. Where does that leave us? For better or worse, it means that you and I must do our best to understand the changes that we see taking place in the health care delivery system, even as they emerge, and we must consider their impact in light of the tremendous amount of information we have available in framing our understandings. Admittedly that is not an easy assignment.

This task is made more difficult by the army of "spin doctors" out there with what appear to be unlimited resources, all aimed at getting the rest of us to accept their respective assessment of the central problem facing the health care system and their preferred solution for solving that problem. This is, of course, not surprising when you consider how high the stakes are and how wide and numerous the competitors range. Don't give up. You are now better prepared to understand the issues than most Americans. You are also likely to find deep satisfaction in using respected sources of information and analytical skills during debates about the successes and failures of our health care system. You will have a much better chance of holding up your end of the argument when you find yourself in debates with persons who rely on ideology rather than real-world facts.

Being able to separate the facts from baseless statements is crucial. So, how can we be certain which "facts" are "factual"? That, actually, is not so hard. Persist in finding out the source of the facts. Who collected the data? Who paid for collecting it? You want to know whether the data collection process is tainted. It might help to keep the tobacco saga in mind. Remember the information the Tobacco Institute put out for years and years before the lawsuits started uncovering documents circulated within tobacco companies?

This book has proceeded from the notion that a sociological framework of analysis is useful in searching out facts that provide the basis for understanding how the health care system came to look the way it does and why change is so arduous. Recognizing that reality can be viewed from different perspectives, which are framed by a larger set of understandings about what one is seeing, should make for more reasoned discourse by reminding us that thoughtful people may look at the same reality and see it differently. This is in contrast to how ideologues see reality. It goes without say that they see reality through their preferred, fixed explanatory frameworks, which they have no intention of altering.

Before we end this discussion, I would like to return to an issue that came up when we first encountered the two sociological perspectives in chapter

2 that we have been relying on throughout the book. While I have maintained that the two perspectives present very different views of reality, it is also true that the two perspectives seem to be in total agreement on a number of critical points. When you think about it, the functionalists maintain that social institutions change when society wants them to change, and that is certainly happening in the case of the health care system. The conflict theorists say that conflict between the haves and have-nots never really stops, and as we have seen, there is good evidence to support that assessment. Given the public-opinion data we reviewed in chapter 3, representatives of the two theoretical perspectives cannot help but agree that society considers this social institution to be less than satisfactory in how it serves us. Where they part company is in their assessment of the predicted outcome. In theory, the functionalists would expect things to improve for all of us, in contrast to the conflict theorists, who would expect the haves to come out ahead, as always. In practice, who could maintain a functionalist perspective, considering the record? There have simply been too few health care system changes over the last few decades that anyone could describe as truly beneficial to the society as a whole.

While I have argued that using a sociological framework of analysis helps to frame the arguments involved so that the problems can be more clearly defined, it is also true that the most sophisticated application of research methods and theoretical analysis will not point to a definitive solution. Science, in this case social science, is neutral with regard to the recommendations regarding actions to follow. This is where policy analysis and decision making comes in. Arriving at some consensus about solutions requires, first, that a substantial number of people see the facts the same way; and, second, that they share a fair amount of agreement on defining the problems those facts point to. Only then can policy analysts go on to identify solutions. However, as you can see, social scientists—even those within one discipline, namely sociology—do not see the world from a single perspective. Considering that similar disagreements plague other relevant disciplines— particularly medical economics but also medical ethics, political science, and public health—defining the problem becomes that much more complicated. Then there are the debates that we considered very briefly regarding the efficacy of various treatments that medical specialists in different specialties are convinced are superior to those being used by colleagues in other specialties. My point is that if medical and social scientists cannot agree, then there is little reason to believe that any large number of people in society will soon be arriving at some consensus. That leaves policy makers without much hope of creating policies that will be welcomed by any significant proportion of the public.

In spite of all the difficulties involved, health and health care are matters too serious to allow misrepresentations of reality to take hold. Do not allow glib representations to go unchallenged. Insist on documentation and facts. Doing so will ensure that the U.S. health care delivery system as a social institution will actually improve rather than simply undergo change. It really is up to each of us—who else?

Just in case you were ready to give up anyway and let the policy makers and other "experts" make the decisions for you, consider the following commentary, offered by a particularly knowledgeable observer. He puts the statements made by one category of health sector participants in perspective by describing the process through which new additions to the health care system come about. The statement, made in 1998, is just as accurate now, perhaps even more accurate.

> The custom among executives in the private health sector is to blame the Health Care Financing Administration (HCFA) [renamed Centers for Medicare and Medicaid Services], as if it were a legislative body, a state within a state, governed by the American analogue of China's Red Guards, which woke up every morning wondering whom next to torment in the defense of a dying ideology. . . . HCFA merely fine-tunes and administers compensation methods that have been concocted as part of that never-ending game between members of Congress and the legions of lobbyists who besiege the Capitol and who busily help Congress write the laws that it passes. If the private-sector executives who chafe under the complexity of government regulation wished to discover the culprits behind the complexity, and if they wanted to be brutally honest with themselves, they would look into the mirror first, look at Congress next, and only then look at the government bureaucrats who administer the laws hatched out by the former two. . . . It would be unseemly to blame these arcane rules on government alone, and it would be truly egregious to blame it on the hard-working HCFA bureaucrats who must convert bewildering legislative effusions into operational rules that are fair to the millions of Americans who depend on Medicare and Medicaid for their health care, fair to the American taxpayer who foots the bill for these programs, and fair to the income-seeking private purveyors of health care who look upon the American taxpayer as their source of fiscal nourishment.[1]

As if the efforts of spin doctors, lobbyists, and others who speak for various interested parties were not enough to hinder our taking a reasonable position about possible changes to the health care system, there is still another set of issues making it difficult to do so—issues that we have not even touched on in the preceding pages. When people begin arguing about the changes that are needed, there is a good chance that someone will ask what it is we are ultimately trying to achieve in pursuing change. When pushed to its logical conclusion, this question introduces a whole set of new issues, which lend themselves to various interpretations, which in turn leads to more debate and argument, and so on.

Throughout this book, we have been so focused on the trees that we did not take time out to look at the forest. To continue this analogy, we did not consider what is responsible for the forest being there in the first place—that is, that huge stand of people who are sick and dying. What factors do you think are primarily responsible for people's health problems and untimely deaths? Do you think that improved access to health care is really the most critical factor in reducing the rate of illness and increasing life expectancy? Or is it that people are causing their own health problems through their bad habits and behavior (smoking, drinking, eating junk food, not exercising)? Or do you think that the ultimate responsibility lie in genetics and biology—genes that make one susceptible to cancer, for example, or the differences associated with gender or race? Then there are the far more complex sociocultural explanations—such as poverty, racism, and an even more complex factor, social inequality—each of which respected researchers have found to be closely linked to variations in morbidity and mortality rates. Why do we have to agree on an answer? Because that answer provides the basis on which appeals are made for the distribution of funds to support efforts that will do the most good. When there is no agreement on what is primarily responsible for illness and death, it is difficult to know where to put the money. Consider the options.

We have spent all this effort thinking about the health care delivery system. But what if that is not the most important factor responsible for the differences we see among people in their illness and death rates? What if personal behavior is really more important? If so, then we should redirect funds from being used to address health problems after they occur, where the majority of funds go now, and instead aim them at preventing problems in the first place. That means increasing funding for public education, programs helping people avoid addiction to cigarettes, alcohol, and drugs, as well as teach them how to improve their diet, prevent accidents, and so forth. If one's health is actually mostly a matter of the genes one inherits, then we should shift a greater proportion of public resources to research on genetic mapping, screening, splicing, and so on. If, however, morbidity and mortality are more closely connected to such multidimensional and difficult-to-grasp factors as racism, poverty, and especially social inequality, then what? Then we must be prepared to make some really big social changes. Most people feel overwhelmed when they consider the implications of taking on the latter agenda. It is just too much—too hard, too threatening, too overwhelming to contemplate for most people. Taking any kind of stance becomes all the more burdensome because of all the work that must go into defining and defending it.

That may be, but we cannot ignore these questions. This does not mean we will now attempt to answer them. They deserve thorough consideration, and that requires at minimum another book-length discussion. (I can recommend a number of books that do exactly that.)[2] I also recognize that we need some closure on the issues we took up in earlier chapters. In short, now that we have gotten a glimpse at the forest, it will be difficult to ignore it in considering the changes we decide to support. Acknowledging that, let's go back to looking at the trees, with the aim of considering what short-run changes we would like to see in the structure of the health care system. That focus brings us back to the underlying question of this book—that is, exactly what is it about the health care delivery system that we want to see changed, and what rationale are we prepared to offer for recommending the solutions we ultimately decide to support?

If you were expecting a fully developed list of such changes from me, you are going to be disappointed. In fact, I find it difficult to get beyond what I see as the single biggest obstacle to moving forward in making any kind of change. Once we confront that, I believe that working out other changes will be easier. In my estimation, the biggest question we as a society face is deciding who should have primary authority over the structure of the health care delivery system. Or, if you prefer, who we want to see in charge of *rationing* health care services. Yes, rationing! Face it: we can't deliver all the health care services all of us might want, so we have to decide how to set limits. The only logical way to do so is to decide whom we are willing to trust to do it.

To whom we decide to give primary authority for making these decisions determines how the restrictions will work and who will bear the brunt of them. The fact that we cannot agree on one or a combination of authorities is what immobilizes us. There are not that many alternatives, basically only three, for establishing a locus of control for making health care delivery decisions. One option is the government, which Americans are convinced is inefficient and incompetent. We must recognize, however, that it is best equipped to ensure fair and equitable access to health care for everyone. Another option is the medical profession, which we no longer trust. Its strength is now, as it has always been, the expertise to diagnose and treat disease and advance medical knowledge that will provide better diagnostic tools and treatments in the future (i.e., quality). The third option is the market approach, meaning competition. Its strength is its ability to apply organizing techniques developed in other sectors of the economy for the purpose of improving organizational efficiency and cost containment. We certainly do not have much reason to think that reliance on market forces has brought us cost containment.

As I have said, I believe that we must come to some consensus about which of the three alternatives or what combination of them we are willing to support before we can hope to pursue specific changes. Personally, I believe that we would benefit most from seeing a little more cooperation and a lot less competition among the major players involved in the operations of the health care delivery system.

In the hope that the following will be constructive in achieving a greater degree of consensus on that very point, I would like to comment on the reasons behind our current state of dissatisfaction with the market approach. In my view, it is not competition per se that is responsible for the high level of dissatisfaction Americans express with regard to our health care arrangements. I agree with the critics who point to something more specific — namely, the degree of organizational disruption that competition invariably brings. We as a society were ready to support competition because we took what the representatives of the corporate sector and many economists said at face value. They said that the special skills that businesspersons were bringing to this sector would make health care organizations more efficient; that, in turn, would dramatically lower costs and increase our choices, both of which would result in our greater satisfaction. However, as we all soon discovered, organizational change, even if it is for the purpose of improving operations, means disruption, which is upsetting when it affects familiar, efficient, and rewarding patterns of interaction, such as the long-standing, gratifying relationships that develop between doctors and their patients.

Patient satisfaction surveys have consistently found that a major source of dissatisfaction is due to patients being unable to select their own doctors. Doctors and other health care workers have traditionally considered established relationships with patients to be an important source of gratification. The fact that competition treats organizational restructuring as a necessary step in the quest for improved efficiency forces doctors and patients to play musical chairs while everyone watches to see whether there will be a place for them as the game continues.

Organizational restructuring causes some doctors to leave, insurance coverage for selected services to change, new procedures for making an appointment with doctors to be introduced, and referrals to familiar specialists to be disallowed. Patients are forced to find a new doctor. It takes time to develop a sense of confidence and trust in the new organization and its doctors, who are, after all, strangers. This raises an interesting question — why is it that we are not willing to give a new doctor a break and extend a little trust to begin with? The answer is apparent in the operating premise in which competition is grounded. Competition assumes "that all are in to get out as much as they can for themselves." That obviously fosters an atmosphere of distrust in the motivations of others and encourages everyone involved to try to outsmart the other guy and get as much for oneself as one can. I have to admit that I do not think that this is an ideal set of values on which to base the workings of the health care delivery system as a social institution. It certainly does not help build gratifying doctor–patient relationships or mutually rewarding working relationships with anyone else in the system.

Organizational disruption occurs because success in a highly competitive environment requires increasing market share (share of customers), which leads to the buying, selling, and taking over of entire health care delivery networks. The organization that beats its competitors risks losing a certain amount of patient loyalty but achieves an enviable stock market profile that translates into impressive financial gains as the stock soars.

In the end, it seems to me that when we look at what the spirit of competition has brought us, it is not at all clear that we as a society ever really wanted efficiency to begin with, especially as we got a closer look at what it meant. I believe that we confused *efficiency* with *effectiveness* and were actually expecting more satisfying arrangements to materialize. Isn't that what we were told to expect and are again being told will be forthcoming from "consumer-driven" arrangements?

In my view, marketplace competition functions as an ideal mechanism for pricing of products—new devices and monitoring equipment, for example. It does not function nearly as well in determining the price of services—any aspect of the course of treatment that starts with a visit to the doctor, history taking, tests, possibly a prescription, plus medical advice. The market depends on comparison shopping and consumer satisfaction. Given all the constraints imposed by insurance plans, how does one arrange to shop for a doctor in the face of an acute health problem? Even if one were prepared to shop, what criteria would one use to select, say, a surgeon? Choose the one who made one feel most comfortable? (How does that relate to skill?) Select the one recommended by friends? (If one's friends chose the cheapest or the closest, how does that help?) In other words, to what extent is shopping for medical services just like shopping for any other service, which is what proponents of market mechanisms and competition would have us believe.

In conclusion, I say that it is too soon to know whether our extended experiment based on market forces and competition has produced any long-term changes that are worth the price we have paid in rising dissatisfaction. That question will be determined with greater certainty at some point in the future. It has clearly altered the way that health care services are delivered. It is also true that we continue to spend far more than do people in other countries. We know that people in other countries spend less and are more satisfied with their health care arrangements than we are. We have a far higher proportion of people who are uninsured than what is true of other countries. Our mortality rates are not as good as those of people in a large number of industrialized countries. But, that's where we started this discussion, isn't it?

NOTES

1. Uwe Reinhardt, "Columbia/HCA: Villain or Victim?" *Health Affairs* 17 (March/ April, 1998): 35–36.

2. Grace Budrys, *Unequal Health, How Inequality Contributes to Health or Illness* (Lanham, Md.: Rowman and Littlefield, 2003); Ichiro Kawachi, Bruce Kennedy, and Richard Wilkinson, *The Society and Population Health Reader*, vol. 1 (New York: New Press, 1999); Richard Wilkinson, *Unhealthy Societies* (London: Routledge, 1996).

Index

About the Author

Grace Budrys is professor of sociology at DePaul University. She also serves as director of the School of Health and Public Service, a unit that brings together professional master's degree programs, including nursing, public services, public health, and social work. Before completing her doctorate at the University of Chicago, she worked in various health care–oriented organizations, including a major teaching hospital, a hospital consulting firm, and a national association dedicated to health education of doctors and patients. Her teaching and research interests have focused on issues related to health organizations and occupations, as represented in two earlier books, *Planning for the Nation's Health* and *When Doctors Join Unions*. Over the last few years, she has turned her attention to the vast disparities in health that exist in the United States, which she addresses in her most recent book, *Unequal Health*.

Breinigsville, PA USA
12 November 2010
249144BV00005B/4/P